NURSING IN LIVERPOOL

SINCE 1862

Nursing in Liverpool since 1862

Meg Parkes
and
Sally Sheard

Every effort has been made to verify all facts in this book but the authors welcome any new information which may not have been available to them at time of going to press.

Nursing in Liverpool since 1862

First published in 2012 on behalf of the authors by
Scotforth Books, Carnegie House
Chatsworth Road, Lancaster, LA1 4SL

ISBN 978-1-904244-85-1

Printed in the UK by Short Run Press Exeter

Contents

'I look to the abolition of all hospitals.
But it is no use to talk about the year 2000.'

Extract of a letter from Florence Nightingale
to Sir Henry Bonham Carter, 1867

Foreword

THIS BOOK is a must read for anybody with an interest in nursing and in particular in the history of nursing and healthcare in the Merseyside region. It sheds light on the past 150 years, charting Liverpool's achievement at the forefront of the development of professional nursing in Britain. The authors draw attention to the passion, diligence and sheer determination of not only our nursing predecessors but also Liverpool's social reformers who paved the way for much that we now take for granted.

The book covers the power struggles and battles that have raged within nursing since the late nineteenth century: everything from the fight for registration to contemporary issues such as standards of nurse education and practice. We can draw direct comparisons with the issues of today on staffing and values such as compassion. Most importantly the values of respect, honesty and dedication are as vital to the profession today as they were 150 years ago.

It takes a special kind of person to be a nurse and this book highlights some very special nurses indeed: individuals who long ago created a legacy for modern nursing as well as a few of the nurses who have trained and nursed in Liverpool over the past 60 years. As nurses we have a lot to be proud of and here in Liverpool we can be proud of our contribution to a nursing legacy that is truly inspiring.

Andrea Spyropoulos
President of the Royal College of Nursing

Acknowledgements

THE AUTHORS would like to thank all those who have contributed to this book: the Royal Liverpool and Broadgreen University Hospital Trust, the University of Liverpool and Liverpool John Moores University for funding; the archivists and librarians at the University of Liverpool's Special Collections, the Liverpool Record Office, the Liverpool Medical Institution, the Royal College of Nursing archives in Edinburgh and both the Nursing and Midwives Council and the Queen's Nursing Institute archives in London.

Sincere thanks go to all the nurses who responded to the appeal for oral history and to Scotforth Books (an imprint of Carnegie Publishing) for their help and guidance in the production of this book.

Introduction

THE IDEA for this book came from the Chief Executive of the Royal Liverpool and Broadgreen University Hospital Trust, Tony Bell, in December 2011. It commemorates a significant landmark in medical history – the 150th anniversary of the opening of the Liverpool Training School and Home for Nurses, the first to be founded outside of London. It was officially opened, in temporary premises, on 1 July 1862. It came into existence through the vision and determination of a Liverpool man, William Rathbone VI. He had the ability not only to see what needed to be done, but the drive to get on and do it. To achieve this he sought the advice and support of Florence Nightingale, and while their collaboration saw the steady improvement in the care and welfare of the poorest in the country, it should not be overlooked that their work began in Liverpool.

A steering group was formed to oversee the celebration of this important anniversary, with representatives from the Royal Liverpool and Broadgreen University Hospital Trust, the University of Liverpool, Liverpool John Moores University, the Liverpool Community Health Trust, NHS Merseyside and the Liverpool Royal Infirmary's Nurses' League. In April 2012 a website was launched with a press campaign to request help from Liverpool nurses past and present in putting together the history of nursing in the city. Meg Parkes, who has a background in both nursing and history research, conducted oral history interviews with nurses from a wide range of specialisms, representing nurse training and practice in Liverpool over the preceding six decades. She collaborated on preparing this history with Sally Sheard, a medical historian who has a long-standing interest in the development of Liverpool's health and healthcare.

The book is not intended to be a definitive history of nursing in

Liverpool. Rather, it is a broad brushstroke over the past 150 years, highlighting the major milestones in the development of professional nursing in Great Britain and in particular shining a light on some Liverpool 'firsts' in the field of nursing practice. It is a story of dedication, innovation and caring.

CHAPTER 1

The foundations of professional nursing in Liverpool

Health and healthcare in Liverpool before 1862

Liverpool's role in the development of nurse training in Britain is an inspiring example of nineteenth century philanthropic endeavour which came out of the town's response to the appalling plight of the sick poor. To understand this achievement it is necessary to look back to healthcare in the previous two centuries. Thomas Bickerton, writing a history of Liverpool's healthcare in 1920, presented a popular perception of the unskilled nurse: *'few anecdotes from the History of Medicine are so well calculated to awaken horror in the minds of the present generation as the sordid story of the unskilled nurse'*. He describes the period from the end of the seventeenth century to the mid-nineteenth as the 'dark period of nursing'.

Like most provincial towns of the period, Liverpool was slow to provide medical and nursing care for those who could not afford to pay for attendance in their own homes. Through the Poor Law, parishes raised funds to provide basic welfare for the 'deserving poor', and from 1834 most recipients were required to enter workhouses. Many of these people owed their pauper status to illness, which stopped them working to support their families. Consequently, workhouses also had infirmaries attached to look after the sickest poor. The nursing in workhouse infirmaries was provided by recovering paupers and a few employed women. They had no formal training, and there was very little medical oversight of their work.

There was, however, a philanthropic movement to provide healthcare for the working classes from the mid-eighteenth century. Alongside the rise of merchants and industrialists, voluntary hospitals were built, and dispensaries opened (to give non-residential medical advice and treatment). Although the effectiveness of these treatments was very limited (and often the sugar pills and coloured potions of quacks offered an equally useful placebo effect), voluntary hospitals offered basic welfare, especially rest and food. Some 35 provincial hospitals were founded in Britain between 1736 and 1779. They relied on public subscriptions for their maintenance and upon the goodwill of local medical men who treated patients for free, in the expectation that it would establish their reputations and they could earn sufficient income from their wealthier paying patients, who were treated and nursed in their own homes.

On 25 March 1749 the Earl of Derby opened Liverpool's first voluntary hospital – the Liverpool Infirmary – on land granted by the Corporation at Shaw's Brow (the site of St George's Hall). It was only the ninth voluntary hospital to be built in Britain, erected for 'those in distress from all parts of the nation and Ireland.' It initially had 30 beds and was funded by subscriptions from the leading men of the town – doctors, ship owners and merchants – who gained prestige from being included in the published lists of subscribers. In return for their annual donation they could nominate a certain number of deserving people each year for either outpatient or inpatient care.

The Liverpool Infirmary was run by a board of trustees with responsibility to oversee the smooth running of the hospital and to attract more funds for improvements. The trustees employed a matron to be responsible for all household matters including the furniture, provisions and conduct of both patients and the servants. According to Bickerton, nurses were employed to 'behave with tenderness to the patients and pay respect and civility to superiors and strangers'. They were regarded merely as servants and endured poor housing, long hours and pitifully low pay. Liverpool Infirmary paid its matron £6 per year and the nurses £4 per year. These women had no aspirations to respectability or a calling to care for the sick. Nursing attracted mainly those of an ill-educated and often undesirable background for whom nursing was just a job. Drunkeness among the nurses and bribery by the patients were commonplace.

The regulations for the Infirmary nurses give an insight into the type of woman employed and the expectations of her. She was forbidden to conceal effects of any patient who died in hospital or to take any

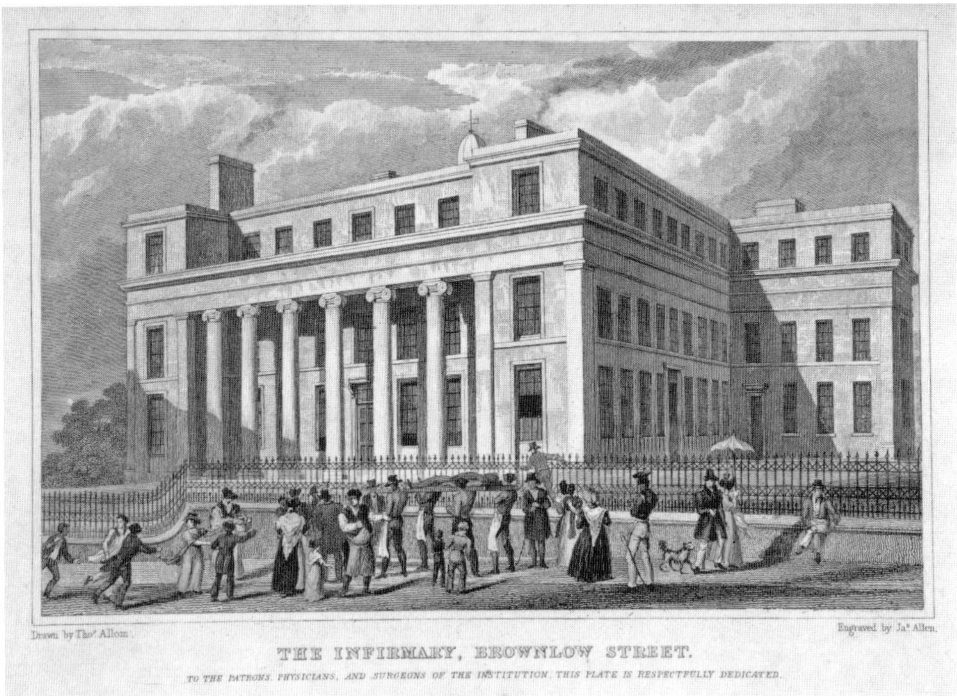

Figure 1.1 *The second Liverpool Infirmary*

fee, reward or gratuity. Dirt and rags were not to be thrown, nor the patients' clothing hung, out of the windows. One window at least in every ward had to be left open night and day. Any nurse concealing the escape of any patient from her ward would be discharged. The final regulation reads:

> That all nurses who disobey the apothecary, secretary or matron's orders, gets drunk, neglects their patients, quarrels with patients or do not cautiously reveal to the officers of the House [hospital] all irregularities committed by patients in their wards (such as drinking, smoking tobacco in wards, quarrelling, destroying medicines or stores, feigning complaints and neglecting their cure) shall be immediately discharged [from] the service of the House.

In 1824 the Infirmary was replaced with a new building, this time sited on higher ground at the top of Brownlow Hill. This was deemed a much healthier location where the air would be more bracing and conducive to recovery. It was designed by John Foster and built in the

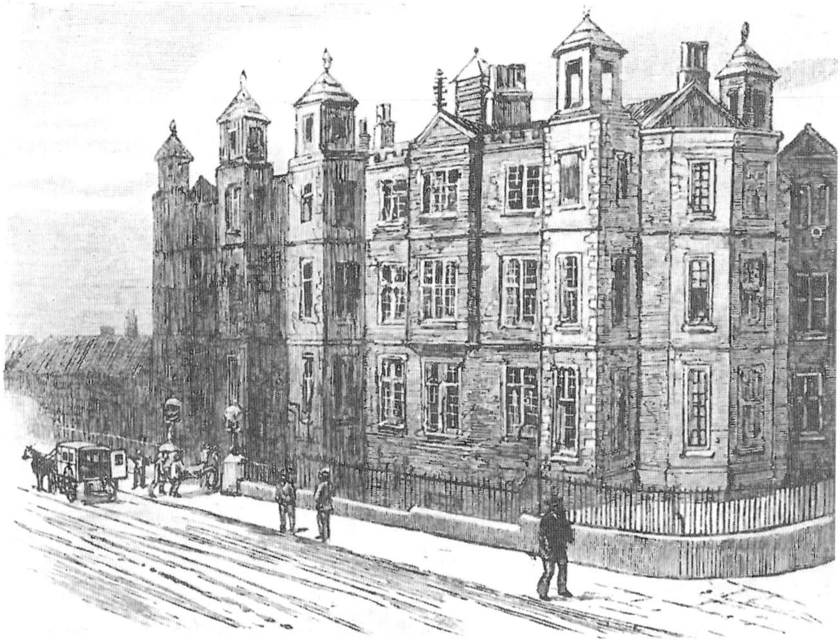

Figure 1.2 *The David Lewis Northern Hospital*

classical style with large, light and airy interiors, believed to be more suitable for a hospital. Following Queen Victoria's visit to the town in 1851 the Infirmary was renamed the Liverpool Royal Infirmary.

On 31 August 1778 Liverpool had opened its first Dispensary at 25 Princess Street for 'such sick and lame poor as were formally in the care of the Parish apothecary'. By 1791 it had moved to larger, purpose-built premises in Church Street, to meet the increasing demand. Forty years later, in 1820, the Dispensary was catering for over 20,000 patients a year. Other hospitals were also opening across Liverpool as the town expanded. On 10 March 1834 the Northern Hospital opened in a house at No.1 Leeds Street. It was specifically to treat men who suffered accidents on the neighbouring docks. After several expansions and moves to different sites, this became the David Lewis Northern Hospital in 1902.

On 17 January 1841 the Southern and Toxteth Hospital opened in Greenland Street, with 30 beds for the treatment of consumption and chest diseases. Over the years more floors and beds were added and in 1857 it was renamed the Southern Hospital. A new larger building opened in Caryl Street in 1872 which became known as the Royal Southern Hospital.

Liverpool led the way in many areas of health and social reform in Britain during the nineteenth century, most notably with the first Public Health (Sanatory) Act of 1846 which created the local government post of Medical Officer of Health. Dr William Henry Duncan (1805-1863) took up this position in January 1847 – the first in Britain. Duncan had been investigating the relationship between poverty, slum dwellings and epidemic infectious diseases for some years. His new role came with the authority to cleanse or close overcrowded and insanitary court and cellar housing. Other new council employees – a Borough Engineer and Inspector of Nuisances – oversaw the municipalisation of the private water companies, the installation of a sewerage system and public baths and washhouses, street paving and cleaning. The poor housing conditions and rise in infectious diseases had been exacerbated by rapid increase in the town's population, with a surge of immigrants arriving from Ireland, especially after the onset of the potato famine in the 1840s. Some had the resources to move on to seek their fortune in America but the majority stayed in Liverpool. This put a huge strain on the town's resources, especially parish welfare relief and the voluntary hospitals.

In 1844 the attention of the Infirmary's Board of Trustees was drawn to the inadequate numbers of nurses: there were only eleven nurses with five assistants to help them, to attend to between 210 and 230 patients. It was also noted that there were no night nurses on the wards. While regarded as very unsatisfactory, it took the Board a further seven years to appoint night nurses and then only four for the whole hospital to work between the hours of 9 p.m. and 6 a.m. In 1853 one young house pupil (trainee doctor), R. J. Banning, noted that nurses were

> *... a very scratch lot, some with practical knowledge but others utterly untrained and mostly slovenly and frequently inattentive... the nurses in the older time were all alike, square-built, stumpy, fat old women, mostly 60 years of age.*

Of one nurse in particular, known as 'Accident Ann' (because she worked in the accident ward) he gives this vivid description:

> *She was the queerest woman I ever saw – had a high well-frilled cap, a bed-gown, linsey-winsey petticoat and large pair of scissors at her side, like shears. She had a most extraordinary walk, waddling like a duck. She wore large shoes, the heels always pushed half-way down.*

Figure 1.3
Florence Nightingale

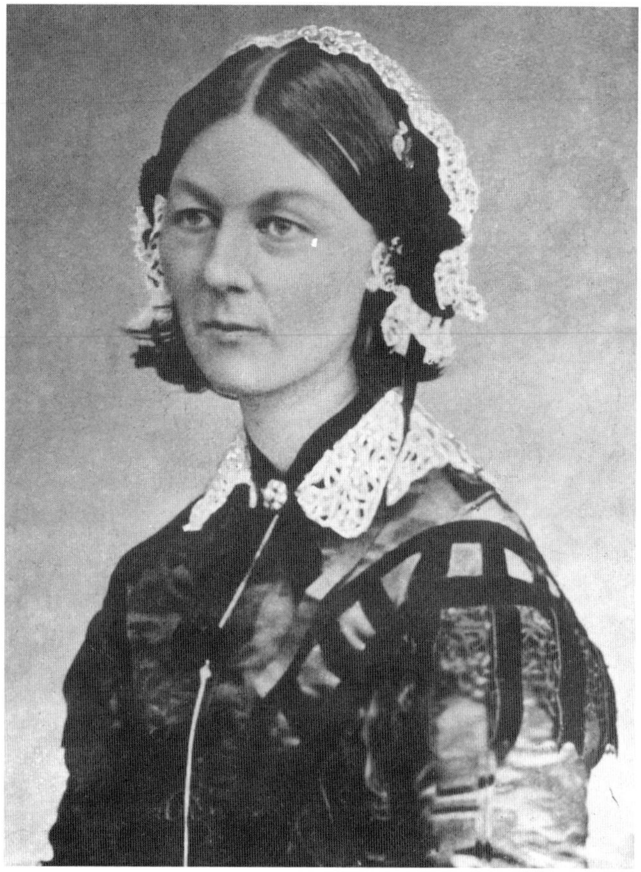

Nightingale, Rathbone and Liverpool nursing

The revolution in nursing in Britain is inextricably linked with the work of Florence Nightingale (1820–1910). Having felt 'called' to nursing as a young woman and against much opposition from her family, Nightingale took a keen interest in how it could be improved and developed. She travelled to Kaiserwerth-am-Rhein in Germany in 1850 to visit the nurse training institution founded there by a protestant Pastor, Theodore Fliedner, in 1836. She returned to Britain determined to emulate this successful scheme. Nightingale's plans for organised training for nurses were interrupted when, in 1854, she was asked to lead a party of British nurses to care for the wounded at the army hospitals in Scutari in Turkey during the Crimean War (1854–1856). The conditions there were appalling and Nightingale worked tirelessly to improve them. On her return she was lauded and a national fund was established in her honour which she used to establish the basis for her life's work, the Florence Nightingale School of Nursing at St Thomas' Hospital in London.

Nightingale used her considerable personal experience of nursing the military sick and injured to influence changes in the practice and perception of nursing. She recognised that nursing had to be of the highest standard in every hospital that claimed to care for and look after the sick. Working almost alone she transformed the standard of nurse training in Britain. Nightingale also used her experiences of the insanitary hospitals of the Crimean War to design a model for a 'hygienic hospital'. Although this was founded on her misunderstanding of how diseases were transmitted (she remained a determined 'miasmatist' – a believer in 'bad gases' – long after the discovery of germ theory), it had a profound influence on hospital design from the 1850s.

There had been earlier attempts at reform of nursing in Britain; the Irish Roman Catholic Society of the Sisters of Mercy (an order founded in Dublin a few years before moving to London in 1839) arrived in Liverpool in 1843 where they founded a House on Mount Vernon and established regular visits to the sick. When Nightingale appealed for women to go to the Crimea to assist her in her nursing work, three of the Sisters of Mercy responded. Two died there and the third, Mary Magdalen Alcock survived and returned to Liverpool. Another initiative, founded in 1848, was the St John's House Nursing Institution. This was a Sisterhood founded by the Church of England for training nurses to work at King's College Hospital in London. Soon after, Louisa Twining (1820–1912), a contemporary of Nightingale's founded the Workhouse Visiting Organisation in 1858 as a means of drawing attention to the conditions, particularly with regard to children and the sick. This later led her to become involved with the issue of trained nurses for workhouse infirmaries and in 1870 she established the Workhouse Infirmary Nursing Association.

In 1849 the newly-married, 30-year-old William Rathbone VI (1819–1902), eldest son of the wealthy Liverpool shipping family, was inspired to get involved in welfare work with the poor in Liverpool. Rathbone was already a noted philanthropist, and in common with the ethos of the day, felt a strong sense of duty to use his wealth and influence for the good of society. He became an honorary visitor for the District Provident Society, collecting savings from poor families, where each week he witnessed the full extent of their misery and appalling living conditions. This was the beginning of his involvement in social welfare work that lasted until his death in 1902.

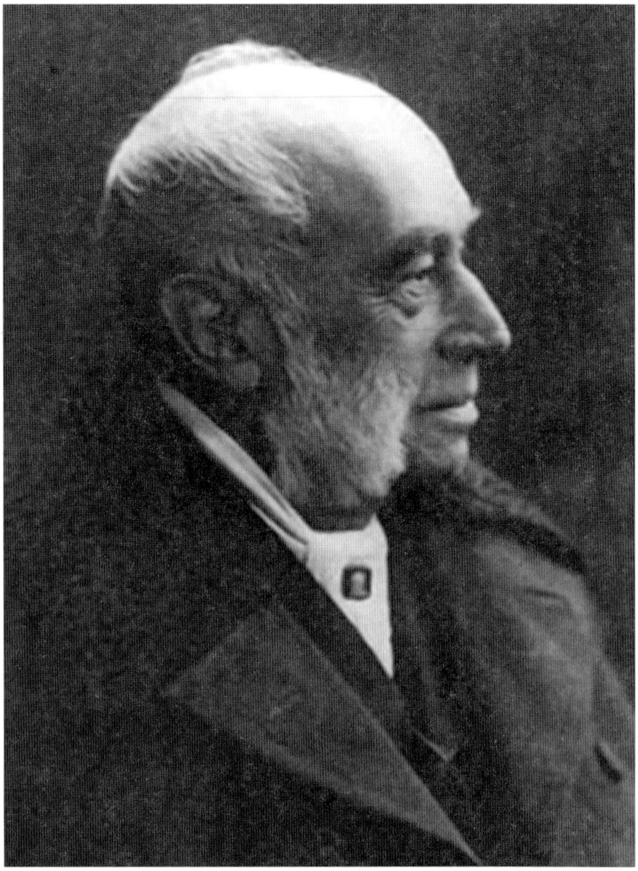

Figure 1.4
William Rathbone VI

In 1859 following the birth of their fifth child, Rathbone's wife Lucretia fell seriously ill and he employed a private nurse, Mrs Mary Robinson, who had trained at the Nightingale School in London, to care for her. He was very impressed by the high standard and quality of care his wife received, especially in light of the stark realities facing the sick poor which he had witnessed at first hand through his visiting work. After his wife's death Rathbone engaged Mrs Robinson for a three-month experiment: he asked her to go out into the neighbouring district to care for and nurse the sick poor in their homes. He could see no reason why the poor, just because they could not afford help when they got sick, should be denied this basic human care. Mrs Robinson agreed but was so overwhelmed by the enormity of the task that within the first month she begged to be released from her contract as she felt unable to continue. Rathbone persuaded her to see it out to the end of the three months by which time she declared that there was nothing,

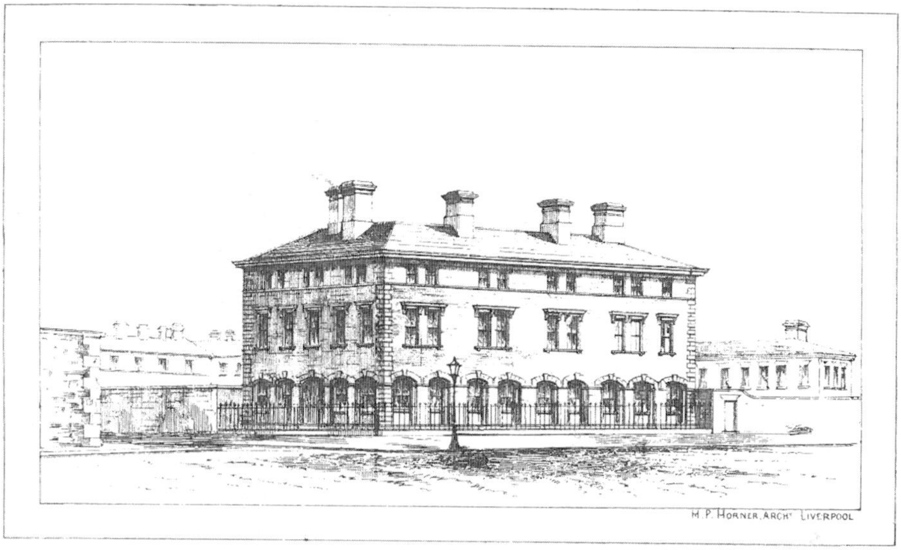

Figure 1.5 *Drawing of Liverpool's first purpose built Training School and Home for Nurses opened in 1863 (from Organisation of nursing in a large town by Florence Nightingale, 1865)*

and nowhere else she would rather be, than working with the sick poor of Liverpool in their own homes. Rathbone was delighted at her decision but realised she would need help if this new 'district nursing' was to become a reality for more than just the needy families within his collecting district.

In the early days of district nursing most of the nurses' work involved providing the sick with the basics, such as nourishing food like broth, clothing and bedding as so many of the poor had nothing. This 'giving of alms' underpinned the work that later developed: instruction in how to clean, wash and feed the sick and proper ventilation of the room. Mrs Robinson quickly saw the results of her work which is why she decided to stay. The sick poor that she tended on a regular basis began to recover and they began to learn how to care for themselves and their families. Rathbone's experiment had worked.

Rathbone turned to the trustees of the Royal Infirmary to ask if they could spare nurses to be trained to become new district nurses. The response was not favourable: because of the demand for nursing work on the wards there were none to spare. There was another problem too. The Royal Infirmary could not train more nurses because they had no space to house the new probationers or undertake the necessary classroom teaching required throughout their training. It came down to a matter of the lack of space. Rathbone wrote to Nightingale for her advice and assistance in making his plan a reality. He needed a supply of qualified nurses but she informed him that as there were insufficient nurses for the wards in London hospitals regrettably there were none spare to send to Liverpool. However, her advice to him was practical and simple: Liverpool should set up its own training school.

With Nightingale's full support and encouragement for his experiment, Rathbone proposed to the Committee of the Royal Infirmary that he would purchase land near the Royal and build a training school and home, if they would agree to run it. He promised that the majority of nurses would be trained for work on the wards at the Royal Infirmary with the rest shared between district nursing of the sick poor in their homes and private nurses for the wealthy. If the experiment failed he agreed to donate the new building to the Infirmary for its sole use.

With such an offer on the table there was no further resistance. Rathbone purchased a piece of land at the rear of the Royal Infirmary on the corner of Ashton Street (off Pembroke Place) and Dover Street and work commenced straight away. The Liverpool Training School and Home for Nurses opened on 1 July 1862 in temporary premises at 56 Bedford Street South while the new building was under construction. It was only the third training school for nurses in the country (the others being at St Thomas' and King's College Hospitals in London) and the first outside London.

Miss Mary Merryweather was appointed as the first Superintendent of the Training School and remained there until 1874. She had been prepared for her role by spending several months in London, sent by Rathbone, observing the methods and practices at both St Thomas' and King's College Hospitals. In the first prospectus for the Liverpool Training School the objectives were clearly laid out:

1. To provide thoroughly educated professional nurses for the Royal Infirmary.

2. To provide district nurses who should attend the poor in their own homes.

3. To provide sick nurses for private families.

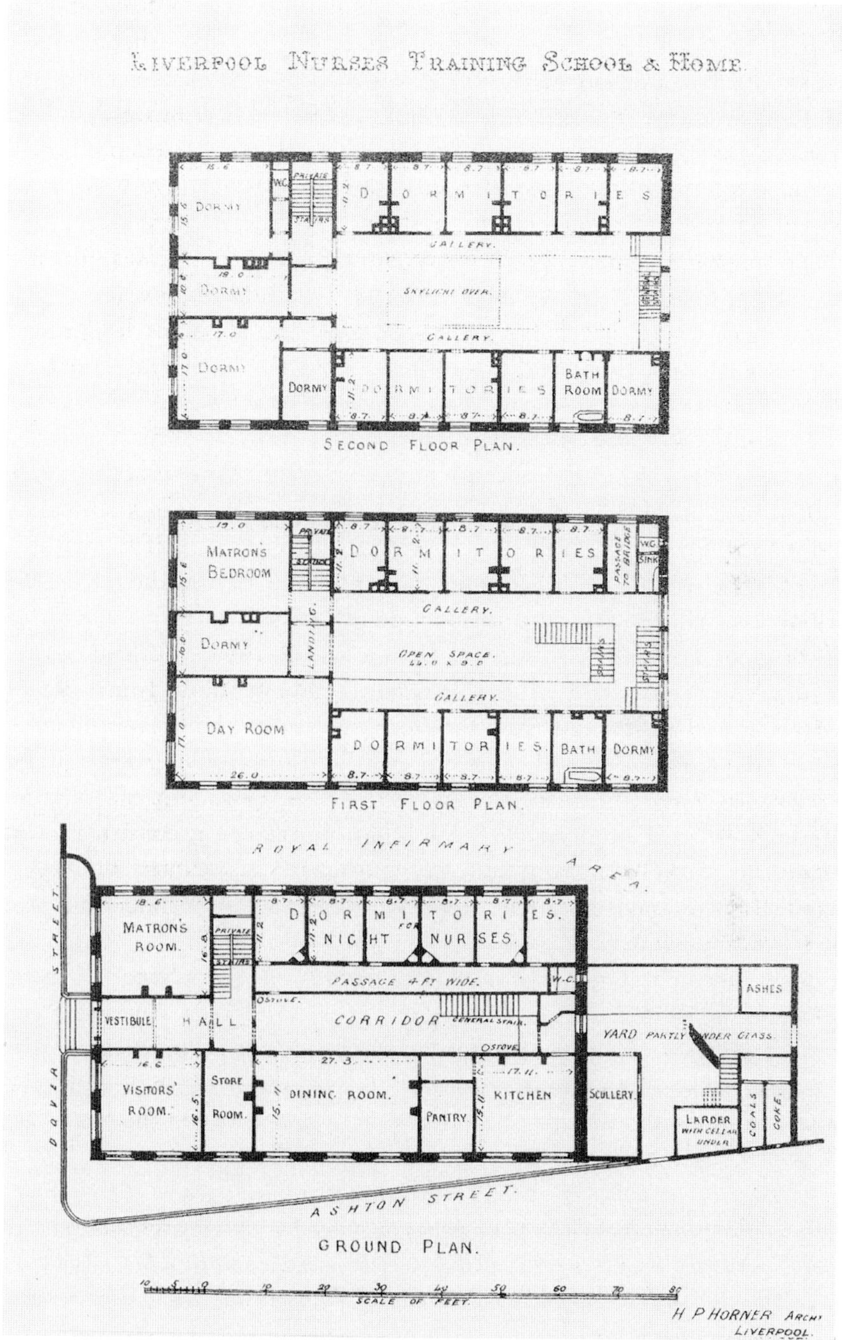

Figure 1.6 *Plan of the interior of Liverpool's Training School and Home for Nurses (from Organisation of nursing in a large town by Florence Nightingale, 1865)*

Now at last Rathbone would have the qualified nurses he needed to expand his pioneering district nursing service. This was to be his life's work and he involved Nightingale in every step of the development and expansion of the Training School and the district nursing service. This support is meticulously documented in the vast collection of letters between the two which has survived. The correspondence shows how Nightingale set out precisely the qualities a nurse should have:

> *Nurses must be real, skilled, experienced… I consider it takes a full year – after the year's training – for a nurse to settle down into efficiency… She has to learn to manage her patients as well as her nursing… to learn neither to be bustling nor overwhelmed when there's a press of work, nor careless when there is none.*

The next problem to address was the appalling conditions found within Poor Law Workhouse Infirmaries, of which Liverpool's Brownlow Hill Workhouse was a prime example. Nightingale had already tried to influence change with the introduction of trained nurses to run these institutions but had had little success due to the tight grip held by the Vestry (the committee of the Parish). Rathbone now joined forces with her and negotiated with the Vestry to allow the appointment of a trained nurse to run the nursing in the Workhouse Infirmary. In 1865 Miss Agnes Elizabeth Jones (1832–1868), a student of both the Kaiserswerth and Nightingale Schools, was appointed as the first Superintendent of nurses at Liverpool's Brownlow Hill Workhouse. However, she had little support and few capable nurses to work with and the task was enormous. Within two years, by then exhausted, she contracted typhus and died. There was no natural successor to step into her shoes and continue the task.

In June 1874, Nightingale wrote to Rathbone about the example that Liverpool had set to others:

> *… at such a place as Liverpool the advantage is that there is an "espirit de corps" or rather "de ville": the leading men know each other: or perhaps one man can lead. The place is not too large for a general superintendence emanating from a centre… is there anything of the sort in London? Is there not the very reverse of these conditions? … what fulcrum is there for any organisation to compare with your nursing organisation at Liverpool?*

Nightingale's aim was to establish professionally trained nurses in every hospital in Britain: women who were well-educated and of the highest

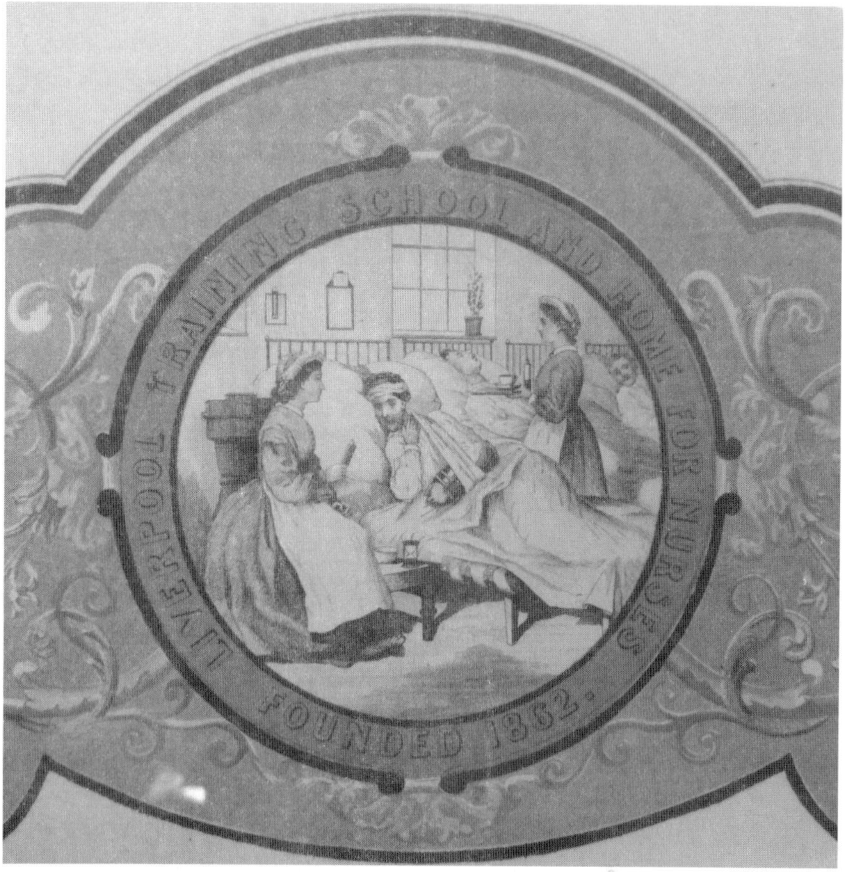

Figure 1.7 *Detail from certificate for long service awarded to Nurse Margaret Sutter on 13 October 1882 by William Rathbone VI, chairman of the committee of the Training School (courtesy of Royal Liverpool and Broadgreen University Hospital Trust archives)*

moral standing, trained to assume complete control of the welfare and care of their patients, and answerable only to the Nursing Superintendent. Rathbone supported her in this work and pursued his own mission to relieve the plight of the sick poor in Liverpool and to encourage others in authority to lead by example that other towns might follow. Theirs was an extraordinary partnership.

Chapter 2

Consolidation of professional nursing

Liverpool's attempts to improve nursing care in the workhouse infirmaries proved successful despite the Guardians' determination to resist change. Though Agnes Jones did not live to see the results of her pioneering work, her diligence and determination to raise standards of care was rewarded and the lives of the sick poor in Liverpool steadily improved over the years. While they would not agree to Florence Nightingale's insistence on teams of trained nurses on the wards, the Guardians acknowledged the benefits of having trained nurses in the Infirmary. There had been a noticeable improvement in the care and recovery of the sick and it was evident that the efficiency of the trained nurses actually saved money. Though there was no obvious successor to Agnes Jones and for a while the development of the system of nurse training in the Brownlow Hill Infirmary was delayed, nevertheless the Liverpool experiment was seen to have worked and was copied elsewhere in the country.

William Rathbone's pioneering work in establishing the principle of nursing the sick poor in their own homes continued apace and the district nursing service developed and expanded rapidly. In 1865 and 1867 respectively district nursing was started in Derby and Leicester, in both cases by nurses who had trained under Agnes Jones at the Brownlow Workhouse Infirmary in Liverpool. In London, in June 1874 the newly-established National Association for Providing Trained Nurses for the Sick Poor set up a sub-committee to explore the need for trained nurses to work in London. Rathbone was appointed chairman and naturally consulted Nightingale on the subject. The Committee appointed as Honorary Secretary Miss Florence Lees, one of her namesake's first probationer nurses.

Nightingale, in reforming nursing in Britain, had been guided by the principle that much suffering was avoidable; she had founded professional nursing not to give women a career but to give the sick a service. Lees was asked to investigate and report back on the state of nurse training in both London's hospitals and in the districts. Nine months later her full report was published and by December 1875 the first Central Homes Training school for District Nurses was founded in Bloomsbury with Lees the Superintendent. Nightingale's main objective was to attract better educated women to train as nurses who would then become the managers of training institutions, thereby raising standards not only practically but also socially as well. Her philosophy of nursing as the natural responsibility of women of high social standing was gathering momentum. When Lees married the Reverend Dacre Craven in 1880 she became an Honorary Inspector of District Nurses and ten years later she wrote *The Guide to District Nursing and Home Nursing*, the profession's first textbook.

In 1887, to mark Queen Victoria's Golden Jubilee, the public donated £120,000. £50,000 was used to build the Royal Albert Hall, and the balance was set aside to endow the Queen Victoria Jubilee Institute for Nurses. Rathbone was closely involved with the founding of the Institute, through his role within the Liverpool District Nursing Association. District nurses qualifying in Liverpool were called Queen's Nurses and the Association provided six month placements for probationers in the city. To celebrate the Queen's Diamond Jubilee in 1897, Liverpool raised funds which were used to extend the provision of district nursing in the town. This led to the founding of the Liverpool Queen Victoria District Nursing Association the following year.

Other members of Rathbone's family were also becoming closely involved with developments in nursing. His second cousin, Emily Lyle, became his second wife in 1862 and designed the badge for the Queen's Nurses. One of the first proud owners of this badge was Rathbone's niece, Miss Rosalind Paget. In 1887 Paget founded the first nursing magazine, *Nursing Notes*, which she managed over the next 50 years. Emily Rathbone took an active interest in her husband's work in the development of nursing in Liverpool, becoming a Lady Superintendent in 1864 and in the early 1890s she championed the call for School Nurses. She followed her husband's earlier strategy, by privately funding a nurse to visit five local schools on a regular basis, treating wounds, sores and other minor ailments, following the advice

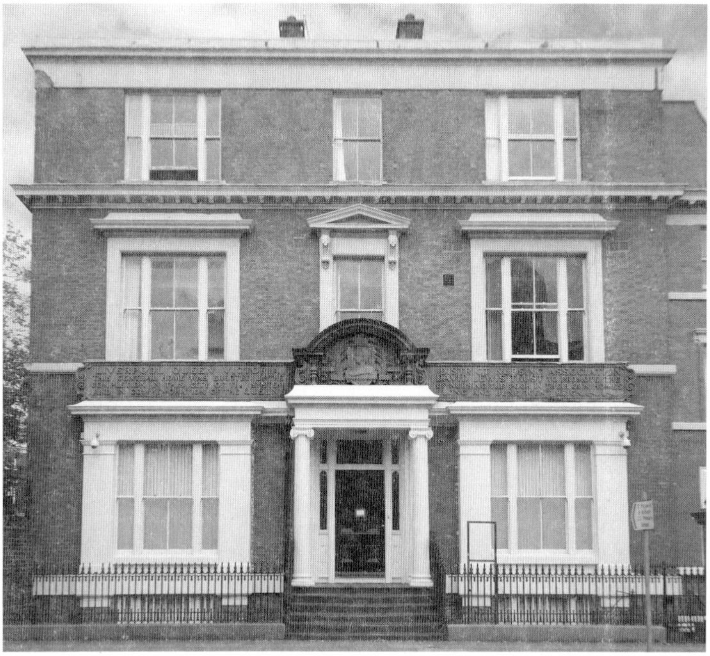

Figure 2.1 *The front of the former Central Home for District Nurses, 1 Princes Road, Liverpool.*

The inscription above the first floor windows reads:
LIVERPOOL QUEEN VICTORIA DISTRICT NURSING ASSOCIATION
THIS CENTRAL HOME WAS ERECTED BY THE DAVID LEWIS TRUST TO PROMOTE THE COMPLETION IN THIS CITY OF THE SYSTEM OF NURSING THE POOR IN THEIR OWN HOMES AND IN COMMEMORATION OF THE QUEEN'S LONG AND BENEFICENT REIGN

of Mrs Leon who had initiated the first school nurse scheme three years earlier in London.

1898 was a significant year in Liverpool, with several healthcare initiatives, including the founding of the Liverpool School of Tropical Medicine, (the first in Britain) and the establishment of nurse training schools at the Northern and the Royal Southern hospitals. In 1900 the trustees of the David Lewis Trust (named after the founder of Liverpool's flagship store, Lewis's Ltd) endowed the new Central Home for District Nurses at No. 1 Princes Road.

This became the administrative centre and headquarters for the Liverpool Queen Victoria District Nursing Association. Nearly 60 years later, in 1959, when the organisation of district nursing was transferred to the Health Department of Liverpool Corporation, the building became the William Rathbone Staff College for the Queen's Institute of District Nursing, the only college of its kind in the world. This eventually closed in 1975 following the reorganisation of the National Health Service.

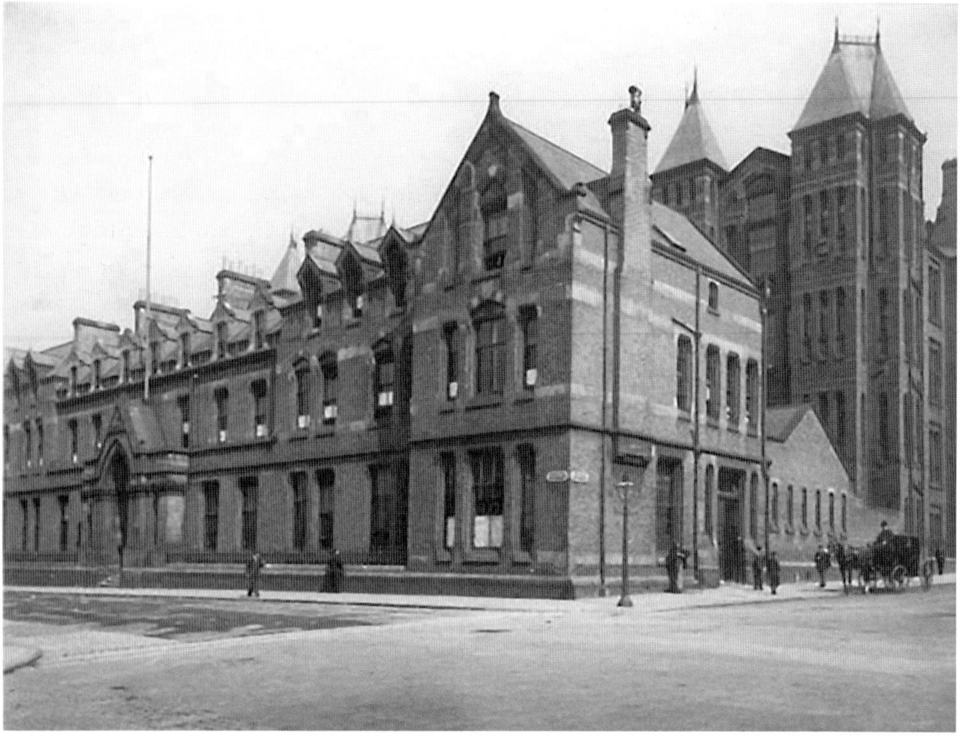

Figure 2.2 *The Royal Southern Hospital*

Early trainees

With the founding of the Liverpool Training School and Home for Nurses, Liverpool Royal Infirmary now had a steady supply of trained nurses to staff its wards. The handwritten register begins with a list of the 20 nurses who were already working at the Liverpool Infirmary on 1 July 1862. They were all transferred to the roll of the Training School. It appears, however, that not all of the applicants for nurse training proved suitable. On the next page in the register the following entries give an insight into the sort of problems Miss Merryweather wrestled with in those early days:

> ***1 August 1862*** *All the night nurses have one after another given notice to leave and their places will taken [sic] with the addition of as few as we can do with. We have engaged one night nurse and only as a temporary arrangement. I. Dickenson – recommended by Mrs Postance, 2 Chesterfield St.*

2 August 1862 *Margaret Ascot came on trial, did not succeed. Elizabeth Craige on trial, she staid [sic] some months but was parted with for supposed untruthfulness and imprudence of conduct…*

The register makes fascinating reading. Subsequent annotations marked out those who were deemed unsuitable for professional training and who were summarily dismissed, often after just a few days or weeks. From the outset the highest standards of personal, moral and professional behaviour were expected. The reasons for dismissal in those early years of the School varied from 'dirty and dishonest' in the case of Annie Rogerson, to 'found totally unfit' as Annie's friend Jackson was described. Mary Mathews, a night nurse, was noted to be 'industrious, but not trustworthy. Parted with for insobriety.' There were others who left early to get married which at the time, and for many decades yet to come, signalled the end of any hope of nurse training. Only if widowed and left in straightened circumstances would married women be considered for nurse training. Twelve years later, three Register entries made between 29 May and 29 July 1874 show that nurses were still being dismissed for being 'not sober'. In 1874 Mary Ann Crane 'left with fever, October 19th'. Nursing was not only morally demanding but also physically dangerous.

Yet despite those who failed to make the grade there were some who complied, worked hard and who must have lived an almost monastic life of devotion to duty and sobriety. These women were eventually rewarded with their certificates and their professional status as trained nurses. The Training School's annual reports have detailed lists of entrants as well as those who failed to make the grade and there was a slow but steady increase in the numbers being trained in the early years. One example is probationer Elizabeth Cooke, whose name first appears in the register when she started training on 7 April 1868. No other personal details are recorded. To the left of her entry is a later annotation reading: Gained certificate 1872. Her name subsequently appears in the 1873 printed Annual Report having received her certificate for three years or more service.

The same principles which had guided the setting up of the first Nightingale Training School for Nurses at St Thomas' Hospital in London in 1861 were rigorously applied in Liverpool, especially character training, the acquisition of skill and knowledge and the principle that nursing administration and instruction was to be firmly in the hands of nurses. Nightingale nurses were trained to go into hospitals and start similar training schemes: they were missionaries who were trained to train.

With the rise in the numbers of trained nurses came improved standards of care and economic efficiency in the running of voluntary hospitals. Combined with the steady increase in medical advances in the treatment of disease from the mid-nineteenth century, hospitals became less feared as 'gateways to death'. The work of medical pioneers such as Joseph Lister with his work on antisepsis, Louis Pasteur in developing pasteurisation, James Simpson in anaesthetics and Robert Koch on bacteriology, all contributed to a greater scientific understanding of health and healing. The wealthy continued to regard hospitals as the province of the sick poor: they entered them only to visit, inspect or govern. Private nursing at home was the preferred option for the wealthy sick until the early twentieth century. However, the public gradually gained confidence in hospitals as places from which the sick could recover and return to normal life. There was growing public expectation in what medicine could achieve. Doctors looked to nurses to administer a wider range of treatments and this in turn brought more patients into the hospitals. In Liverpool, the Royal Infirmary, as the elite voluntary hospital, was regularly at its capacity.

Hygienic hospitals

Florence Nightingale pioneered the need for a radical change in the way hospitals were designed after her return from the Crimea in 1856. As well as her first hand experience during two years of war, she also drew on her considerable knowledge gained from visiting many hospitals in Britain and in Europe in the early 1850s, which gave her an insight into the management and nursing requirements of different types of hospitals.

Nightingale believed that the 'pavilion' style of hospital, as exemplified by the Lariboisière Hospital in Paris, was the best approach to nursing the sick. This advocated long wards built parallel to each other (soon to be known universally as 'Nightingale' wards) running off a central corridor, designed to reduce the risks of cross infection. Each ward had full length windows a bed's width apart allowing the interiors to be flooded with natural light and, more importantly, with plenty of fresh air. Heating was provided by open fires. The ward blocks were separated by open spaces, set out as gardens. If space allowed, single

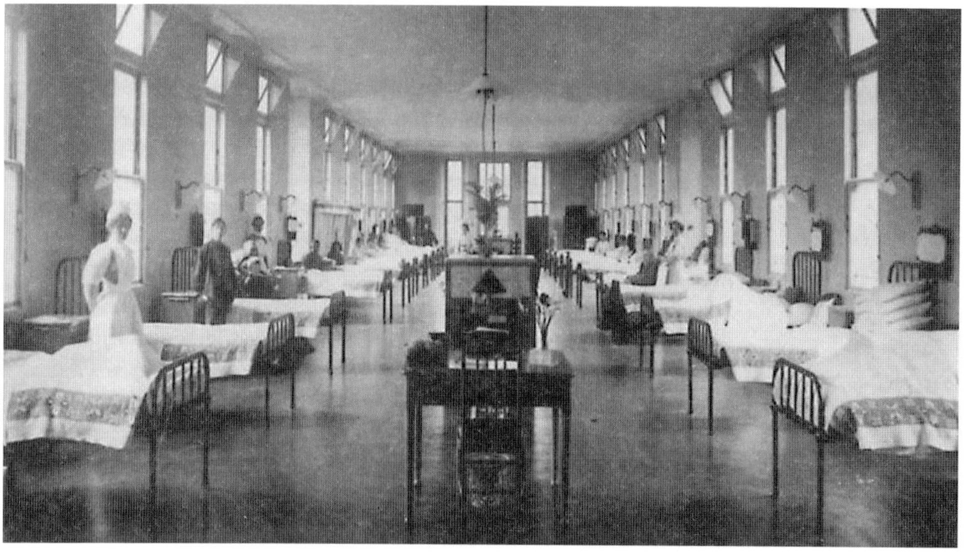

Figure 2.3 *A Nightingale ward in the early twentieth century*

storey ward blocks were the ideal but if an upper floor was necessary the ceiling height should be a minimum of fifteen feet.

Nightingale consulted widely as she developed her plans for the 'hygienic' hospital. In addition to the advising on the ward layout and construction, she also gave instruction on suitable building materials that were easy to clean, heating, sanitation, plumbing, re-siting of cess pits away from wards and the installation of drains and sewers to take waste matter away from the building. She published her *Notes on Hospitals* in 1863 as well as articles in *The Builder* (an influential new trade magazine for architects and the construction industry), medical journals and newspapers. Nightingale was a firm believer in the miasmatic theory – that all diseases were caused by 'bad air', polluted by noxious gasses emanating from the dirty urban environment, and especially cesspits and drains. This underpinned her demands for large windows and lots of fresh air in the wards. Yet there was growing evidence that specific diseases had unique causes. John Snow, through an ingenious bit of early epidemiology, proved that the cholera outbreak in London in 1854 was spread by contaminated water, not through the air. Slowly through the second half of the nineteenth century a new theory of disease transmission took hold – germ theory. Nightingale, however, remained a firm miasmatist until her death in 1910.

Nightingale's first priority had been reform of the Army Medical

Service. Her experience had taught her this was woefully inadequate for caring for sick and wounded soldiers. She insisted that trained nurses were essential to the running of the service in peacetime and gave detailed written evidence to the Royal Commission on the Sanitary Condition of the Army. A new army hospital at Netley near Southampton was then in the early planning stage and she campaigned against both its site (on marshy ground on the banks of Southampton Water), and the design, which she insisted ought to be constructed on the pavilion plan. Despite her many recommendations the plans for Netley remained largely unaltered. However, Nightingale consulted widely with leading architects and sanitary engineers of the day and used every opportunity to continue publishing her findings.

The new Liverpool Royal Infirmary

In the mid-1860s Liverpool's forty-year old Royal Infirmary was struggling to cope with the demands of an expanding population. Situated at the top of Brownlow Hill, in what was deemed a healthy climate away from the town centre, the Royal Infirmary was by now an integral part of the 'medical quarter' of the town: to the rear was the new Training School and Home for Nurses and nearby were the Lock (STI) and the Lying-In (maternity) hospitals, and the Lunatic Asylum. In 1844 the Royal Infirmary's School of Medicine, a purpose-built institution, was erected on the opposite side of Dover Street, conveniently close for the trainee doctors who were instructed on the wards of the Infirmary. Despite the presence of trained nurses to run the wards and the consequent improvements in standards of care, overcrowding and the limitations of the once fine Georgian building, was a serious concern. It took another twenty years, however, before a replacement was opened. At a town meeting in December 1882 a building fund was launched to fund a new Royal Infirmary, the third to be built in Liverpool in 137 years. The proposal was for a much larger infirmary with up to 290 beds, to be built on an extended site including the existing hospital. It involved the purchase of the majority of the adjacent properties bordering Pembroke Place and Brownlow Street, which took some time to procure.

The architect chosen to draw up the plans and oversee the whole project was Liverpool-born Alfred Waterhouse (1830–1905) who by the 1880s had offices in London. He was at the height of his career, renowned for his high Victorian Gothic Revival style and had a

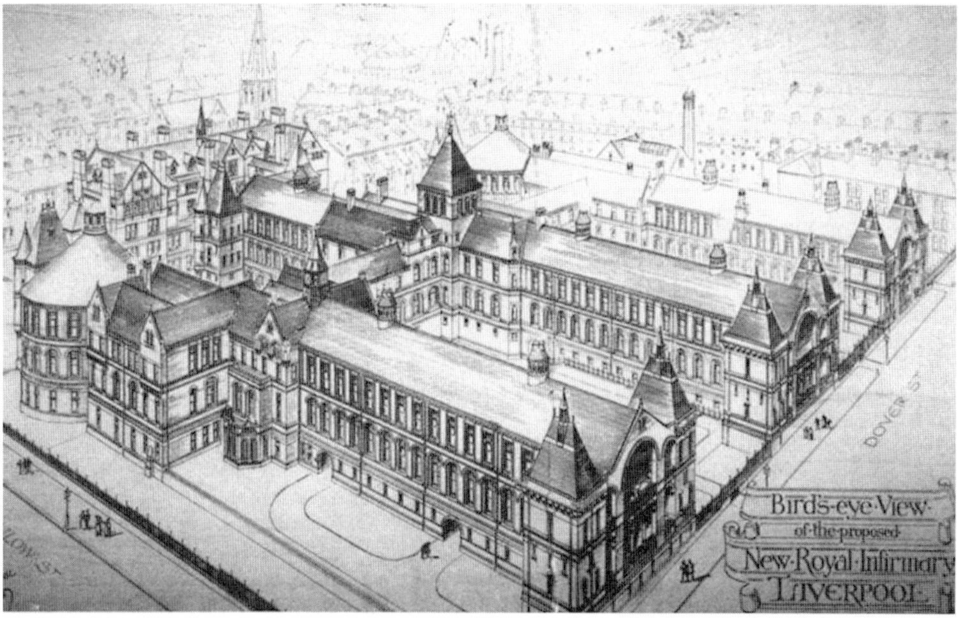

Figure 2.4 *Bird's Eye View of the new Royal Infirmary*

catalogue of important civic buildings to his credit including London's Natural History Museum, several colleges in Oxford and Cambridge, St Mary's Hospital and the new Owens College in Manchester. Closer to home he had designed the North Western Hotel in Lime Street (now home to Liverpool John Moores University students), the Prudential Assurance Buildings on Dale Street, and the Chemistry Laboratories in Brownlow Street. Waterhouse accepted the commission and within days had drafted five possible plans for consideration. He visited many hospitals around the country and consulted widely, including Nightingale, who he invited to comment on his plans which were based on the pavilion plan. She made many suggestions, some of which Waterhouse readily incorporated, such as the number and size of windows, ceiling height, fireplaces in every ward and open spaces between each ward block. However, she did not approve of his use of circular wards, first seen in Antwerp Hospital, as she felt the layout did not allow for sufficient movement of fresh air. On this point she was overruled. Waterhouse had to be pragmatic, on such a limited site he could find no other way to provide the number of beds required.

The new Liverpool Royal Infirmary was opened on 13 November 1889. It had taken two years to build and had run £61,000 over the original budget of £120,000. However, it featured many state-of-the-art innovations, such as glazed brick interiors, allowing for ease of regular and thorough cleaning. The floors were of the latest, patented fireproof materials and there was steam heating throughout the hospital. The high ceilings advocated by Nightingale, combined with Waterhouse's use of glazed and patterned brick archways in the corridors, gave a sense of magnificence to the interior. There were stables for the horse-drawn ambulances and a beautiful chapel for the patients and staff. The hospital was like a cathedral to health, wellbeing and learning, a building fit for the very best in medical care. The remaining properties on the corner of Pembroke Place and Brownlow Street eventually became available and in 1909 a new Outpatients' Department was commissioned. By this time Waterhouse had died and another Liverpool architect, James Doyle (1840–1913), drew up sympathetic plans to mirror the original hospital. This department opened in 1911.

The struggle for nursing registration

Against this backdrop of change and improvement in healthcare in Liverpool there was growing concern nationally about the status of nursing in society and, in particular, in hospitals. The question of registration for nurses had been discussed for some time. Medical practitioners had been licensed since the creation of the General Medical Register in 1858, which helped to standardise their training and qualifications. In 1892 Liverpool Infirmary's Medical Board was drawn into the centre of the argument when Mr Wainwright wrote from St Thomas' Hospital requesting that Liverpool oppose the setting up of a College of Nursing. This new body was intended to oversee the registration of nurses.

There were two types of nurses: the lady-pupils who were from the upper strata of society and who paid to undertake one year's training and then there were the probationers who were paid a modest salary for a training that could take up to four years to complete. There was confusion: the quality of nurse training varied considerably and often the wealthy patient could not easily discern the capabilities or qualifications of the private nurse.

Florence Nightingale had made it clear from the 1850s that she did not want registration for nurses. Some accused her of seeking to cling on to her authority but she strongly believed the qualities necessary to make a really good nurse could not 'be tested by public examination, though it may be tested by current supervision.' Her concerns were to protect the practical skills and learning acquired in ward work and not to fix the standard of training at such an early stage in the development of professional nursing as by doing that, in time it might prove to be too low. Nightingale chose not to publicly state her views preferring to use her considerable influence and authority to steer the debate from behind the scenes. When the issue arose she turned to St Thomas' Hospital for their support. They in turn requested that Liverpool Infirmary also oppose the plans. Liverpool agreed. The ensuing battle for registration was set to last for almost 30 years, 'a battle for status conducted against a background of rampant snobbery and militant feminism', as Abel-Smith put it in his history of nursing. Opposing organisations flourished.

Henry Burdett (1847-1920), who was spokesman for the Hospitals' Association, supported the idea of a central registry but only as a source of information to aid Lady Superintendents and doctors in checking the suitability of nurses applying for jobs. In 1887 he called a meeting of leading nurses including the superintendent of Great Ormond Street Hospital, Miss Wood, and Mrs Bedford Fenwick. Fenwick was outspoken and strident. She had trained in Nottingham and risen quickly in the nursing profession and in 1881, aged 24, had become matron of St Bartholomew's Hospital (Bart's) in London. She represented the militant lady-pupils who like herself, came from the upper echelons of society. These nurses took on organisational roles and responsibilities within hospitals after their one year training.

Fenwick insisted that the highest standards could only be achieved in nursing by employing young women from the higher social classes. She supported registration as a way of controlling the intake into nurse training by stipulating fees for training and examinations geared to the better educated. Not afraid to use scaremongering tactics among her own class she undermined private nurses, stating that without registration there was no control over those who had some training but were found unfit: 'They go into prison, they come out again, they go on nursing.' She sought parity with the medical profession for nurses, as a means of aspiring to positions of greater prestige within the hospitals and in society. She espoused the cause of the suffragettes, was an admirer of Mrs Emmeline Pankhurst and was a formidable force to be reckoned with.

Once aware of Burdett's proposals, Fenwick withdrew from the meeting taking with her many of her supporters. They reconvened and set up the British Nursing Association, its main aim being the registration of nurses, in what was a direct challenge to Burdett's Hospitals' Association. The BNA had a large General Council of over 300 medical and nursing representatives, with Fenwick as its permanent President surrounded by her staunch supporters. It sought to keep power in the hands of the matrons and doctors of London's teaching hospitals, to the exclusion of their counterparts in the provinces who were completely unrepresented on the General Council. The BNA established its own Register which, in keeping with its aims of keeping standards high, was to be only for lady-pupils with just one year's training prior to 1 January 1889. Thereafter the BNA decreed that eligibility to join the Register would require the new compulsory three year training with, of course, its annual fees. This effectively restricted applicants to middle and upper class women. They also tried to standardise training nationally but in this they were not successful. However, their argument that extending nurse training for all to three years would bring stability to the wards of the large training hospitals was eventually endorsed and taken up nationally in 1889.

Nightingale, however, still had great influence with many of the matrons around the country who, in turn, would carry their nurses with them. Interestingly, the strongest opposition to registration came from the matrons of both of the London hospitals where Fenwick had worked: the London Hospital and St Bartholomew's. Both matrons believed the proposed registration would narrow the field for recruitment and cause staff shortages on the wards, excluding 'many women who would make excellent nurses.'

There were many factions. The provincial and rural medical establishment, represented by the Incorporated Medical Practitioners Association, saw registered nurses as a threat to their livelihoods, competing for work with the sick who had a growing respect for nursing. The British Medical Association represented doctors in the metropolitan and provincial teaching hospitals who understood the value of competent nurses to whom they could entrust the delivery of ever-more complicated treatments. There were matrons who believed that registration would enhance their personal standing, and there were those who were afraid that regulating nurse training schools would find their own institution wanting. Against this backdrop, in the early twentieth century the role of women underwent a radical change. They began to demand respect, a purpose and a role in society. For many young women, from all strata of society, nursing had become a respectable and honourable profession, a means of casting off the shackles of boredom or duty to Mama or, in the case of those below stairs, servitude to the 'master'. It was an unsettling time which saw many private feuds and rivalries played out on the public stage.

In 1893 the British Nursing Association gained Royal support, enabling this powerful moniker to be added to its title. There were two ways to get registration for nurses: either by Act of Parliament or by Royal Charter. With the support and extensive lobbying by Nightingale's staunch ally William Rathbone VI, now an MP, the first route was effectively blocked to the Royal British Nursing Association (RBNA). However, it could apply for a Royal Charter to enable it to register nurses. The Privy Council did grant a Charter but it fell short of expectations. It was suspected that once again Nightingale's influence had secured a vital change in the wording, substituting 'list' for the word 'register'. The Charter also radically altered the composition of the General Council no longer allowing for a permanent President. This seriously hampered the ambitions of the Fenwicks: in 1894 Mr Bedford Fenwick resigned as treasurer of the Association, followed by his wife later that year. However, they quickly regrouped and founded a splinter group, a private nurses' society and then soon afterwards the Matrons' Council of Great Britain and Ireland, which represented those matrons who supported the registration of nurses.

In 1896, with the Charter and its 'list' falling well below the Royal British Nursing Association's expectations and the aggressive and critical tactics of the Fenwicks, the Association passed a resolution opposing the state registration of nurses. By the turn of the century doctors were divided about the merits of registration. Provincial medicine, largely represented by the Incorporated Medical Practitioners Association, felt threatened by the prospect of registered nurses becoming a rival for public esteem, and more importantly, fees for services. Yet the London hospitals had no shortage of nurses applying to train in them, unlike in the provinces where training schools were competing for the right calibre of applicants.

In the end, the impetus to resolve the issue of registration came from the example set first by the teaching profession which in 1899 was granted registration for all levels of teachers. This was closely followed in 1902 by an Act of Parliament which created the Register of Midwives. In the same year the Society for Registration of Nurses was founded and in 1904 this amalgamated with Fenwick's Matrons' Council with the common purpose of securing state registration for nurses. This re-energised the RBNA which once again took up the cry. Repeated Select Committees were convened to hear arguments from all parties and rival Registration Bills were placed before Parliament. In 1905 a Select Committee voted in favour of establishing state registration for nurses and appointed a Central Body which was to keep the Register, admitting all those who had had 'approved' training including existing nurses who could provide evidence of efficiency and character, and an approved standard of training schools. It was intended that after four years this body would report to the Privy Council on whether a separate Register for nurses trained to a lower standard should be created. This last requirement took nearly forty years to come to fruition.

With these constant delaying tactics, frustration grew. This resulted in a conference of all parties which established the Central Committee for the State Registration of Nurses. In 1910 another obstacle to progress was removed with the death of Florence Nightingale. With her died the influence that she had so resolutely used to further her own strongly held beliefs. But it was the outbreak of the First World War in 1914 that finally brought the sequence of Parliamentary Bills to an end. The war effort now brought many thousands of women on to the wards of Britain's hospitals, many as members of the Voluntary Aid Detachment (VAD). Other recruits were middle and upper class women who wanted to be of use. It was an intoxicating mix and it stirred professional nurses, irrespective of previous allegiances, to finally band together in protection of their training and their status within hospitals. In 1916 a proposal to form a College of Nursing came from a new quarter, the combined forces of the Army Medical Board, the Head of the British Red Cross Society and former matron of Guy's Hospital and the Chairman of Joint War Committee of the British Red Cross Society and Order of St John. Their recommendation rapidly gained support as none of the protagonists had been publicly involved in previous battles within nursing and in March 1916 the College of Nursing was established. While the College did not directly advocate the registration of nurses nevertheless it pointed out the advantages to the profession of having leadership and organisation. It was quietly diplomatic, had no axe to grind or vested interests but at the same time had many influential supporters. By June 1919 two separate Bills had placed before Parliament. With no resolution to either, the Minister of Health, Dr Christopher Addison, stepped in and urged the Government to bring its own Bill. In December 1919 the Registration of Nurses Act was passed. This created the General Nursing Council to oversee the State Registration of Nurses.

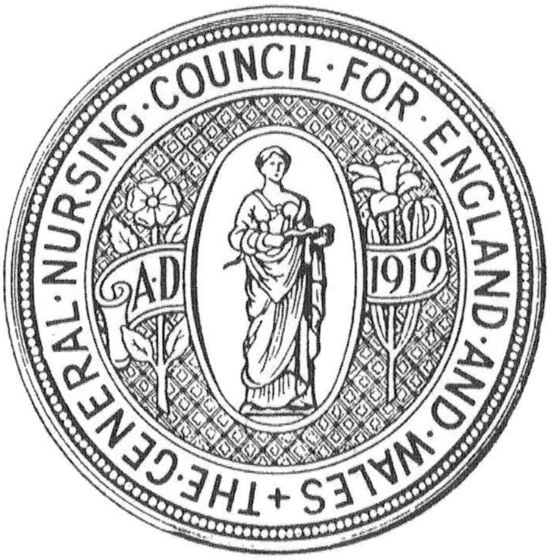

Crest of the General Nursing Council created in 1919 (courtesy of the Nurses and Midwives Council archives)

A combination of the effects of the women's movement, the need to do one's duty for the war effort, professional integrity and protectionism and the establishment of the College of Nursing – an organisation unfettered by decades of argument and disunity – finally brought about registration. The war may have been won, but the battle to establish professional nursing was set to continue.

CHAPTER 3

1919–1948: From registration to the start of the NHS

THE INTER-WAR PERIOD provided a battleground, this time for the opposing sides in nursing. This chapter examines the consequences of the fight for registration; the changes in the organisation of hospitals and healthcare to meet the demands of both the population and advances in medical science; the impact of the Second World War on the development of the nursing profession and the creation of the National Health Service.

The College of Nursing was founded by influential nurses during the First World War. Nursing historian Brian Abel-Smith judged it 'unashamedly elitist'. In advocating a longer training period for nurses it sought to attract young ladies from upper middle class families with a good education. Probationers would be required to sit hospital entrance exams in addition to the national final examinations. From the outset, the College of Nursing sought to exclude from membership of its General Nursing Council (GNC) matrons of small and special hospitals as well as the Poor Law infirmaries, thereby denying representation to a large section of nurses. The nurses from such hospitals were generally considered to be relatively ill-educated and largely poorly-trained.

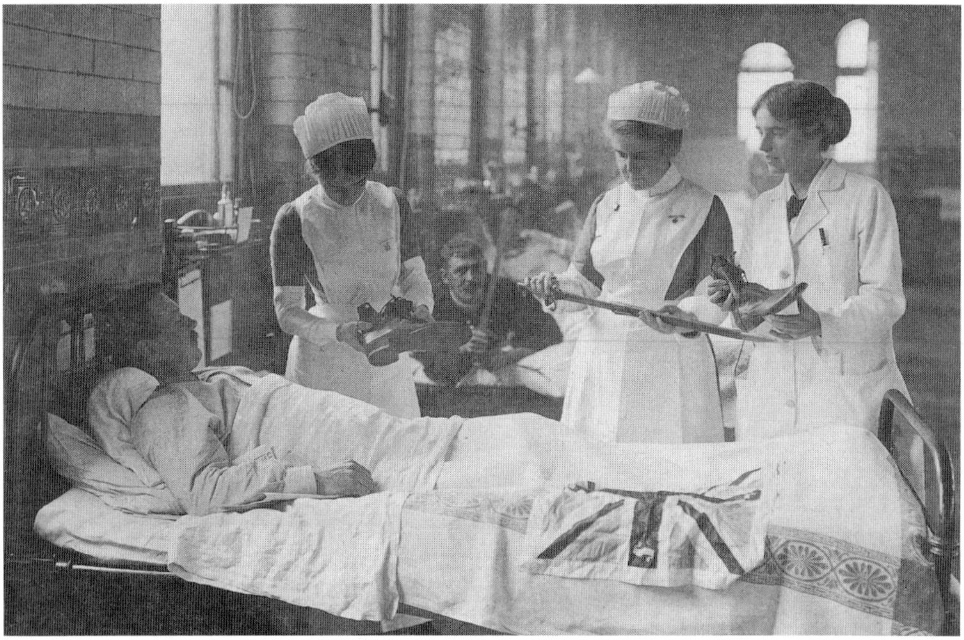

Figure 3.1 *At the bedside of a First World War soldier, 1916, Liverpool Royal Infirmary (courtesy of Cynthia O'Neill, More Pictures of Health)*

Impact of the Voluntary Aid Detachment

At the end of the war most of Britain's larger hospitals were well staffed but this situation did not last for long. Thousands of women had answered the call to serve their country and volunteered under the Voluntary Aid Detachment Scheme – they became known as 'VADs' – run by the British Red Cross. In addition to taking jobs in private nursing homes and the small infirmaries and hospitals across the country, thousands of these volunteers also trained and worked in military hospitals and First Aid posts abroad. As the armed forces were de-mobilised, many of the VADs returning to civilian life looked to nursing for employment. But professionally-trained nurses were threatened by the spectre of this influx of unqualified women 'posing as nurses' as they saw it. Despite the fact that many professional nurses did not support the College of Nursing's campaign for registration, the profession quickly closed ranks against what they perceived was this more immediate threat to their status in hospitals. They were determined that untrained women and in particular the VADs, irrespective of their war service, would not be permitted to take up full time jobs in hospitals at the expense of qualified nurses and certainly should not be allowed to register as nurses.

Compiling the Register

The Registration of Nurses Act in 1919 enshrined the principle of a 'one portal' entry, meaning that only those women who had at least three years formal training would be admitted to the Register. There were six sections to the Register: the General section was only open to females; the male section was for nurses who looked after men with venereal disease; there were specific sections for children's nurses, fever nurses, mental nurses (who were mainly male) and there was a separate section for mental deficiency nurses. As men could not join the General section of the Register they were automatically excluded from election to membership of the General Nursing Council. Nurses who trained in one part of the Register and later wanted to work in another discipline had to re-train for two years, irrespective of their previous seniority and experience. This was one reason why some nurses did not seek to join the Register.

In 1920 the first General Nursing Council (GNC) of the College of Nursing was appointed and charged with starting the Register. The first members of the Register were then required to vote to elect the second GNC two years later. However, the GNC was deeply divided from the outset. The main problem was deciding how to determine the eligibility of 'existing' nurses to join the Register. They identified three categories of nurses: 'existing' nurses who were in the profession before 1919, nurses who had completed their training after the Act, and those who entered after the Act and who would have to sit an examination.

For existing nurses it was decided that the essential criteria for admission to the Register was to be a minimum of one year's training in what was classified as an 'approved' hospital. Hospitals that were approved by the GNC were generally the prestigious 'voluntary' hospitals. Thus for the well-bred and educated lady-pupils – which naturally included Ethel Fenwick and her supporters – registration and eligibility to sit on the GNC, was guaranteed. However, other 'existing' nurses who could prove long service as practical nurses, be that in nursing homes, small specialist hospitals, the workhouse infirmaries or as district nurses, and who had often been trained by highly qualified nurses, had to also provide evidence that they were in practice both in 1919 and also prior to 1 January 1900, in other words for over 19 years. Failure to comply, coupled with their training having not taken place in an 'approved' hospital, meant they were ineligible to register. Training schools were not required to be 'approved' prior to the Act. However, the one-year rule did conveniently deny access of VADs to the Register, which was the intention. The whole system was clearly unfair and weighted against nurses from lower down the social scale, even though they could prove years of competent and dedicated service.

The matter was resolved just before the deadline for registrations in July 1923, thanks to the intervention of the Ministry of Health, the House of Commons and to an amendment tabled by Dr Chapple which broadened the criteria through which many of the 'existing' Poor Law nurses and district nurses could apply for registration. This would now be on the basis of certificates provided by a matron of a general hospital, or two medical men, testifying that the nurse had worked for not less than three years prior to 1919. In the event only around 40,000 registrations were received, far short of expectations, but it quickly became apparent that nurses who were registered stood a much better chance of taking up appointments than those who were not.

Shortage of nurses and recruitment

During the early 1920s the shortage of nurses, particularly in the smaller infirmaries, was a great concern, with articles and comment regularly appearing in the press. To meet demand some smaller provincial hospitals took girls who were too young to apply to training schools to increase the numbers on the wards, and Poor Law unions found it very difficult to attract sufficient trained nurses. In Liverpool, there was a clear hierarchy among hospitals offering general training: middle class respectable girls were actively sought by the Liverpool Royal Infirmary (LRI) where, despite stringent entry requirements, having attended the 'right' school, i.e. a grammar school, or being from the 'right' type of family was often sufficient. Interestingly, while Liverpool was home to large communities of both Welsh and Irish families, the Royal actively recruited among the Welsh but did not encourage applications from the Irish. However, in the Poor Law hospitals, like Smithdown Road and Walton hospitals, not only were Irish as well as Welsh girls welcomed but entry criteria for training were very much lower and, at times of severe staff shortages, could even be waived. This 'segregation' in recruitment also applied to applicants from further afield: the Royal

Infirmary sought applicants predominantly from the south of England while other voluntary hospitals in Liverpool such as the David Lewis Northern and the Royal Southern attracted mainly local girls. Not surprisingly perhaps the nurses had a reputation among the local hospitals for regarding themselves as 'a cut above the rest', no doubt in part encouraged by the upper class aspirations and professional protectionism of its nursing and medical hierarchy.

Traditionally nursing had been seen as an occupation which provided women with a home and a modest income, a vocation for the single or widowed: married women were regarded as undesirable. Before the First World War there had been a rapid expansion in the number of trained nurses. This was partly in response to the system of medical care improving along with a general rise in the standard of living. But in the 1920s voluntary hospitals faced a real crisis, not only because of a dramatic drop in the donations upon which they depended but also by the rise in costs. This was due in part to the legacy of the war but also to the rising numbers of the middle classes who now wished to be treated in hospitals. Older people were still wary of hospitals but the younger generation was much more accepting and confident in the prospect of discharge from, and not certain death in, hospital wards, and wished to have access to new technology such as x-rays and ECGs.

Private patients

One income stream that voluntary hospitals benefitted from was providing private nurses to care for wealthy patients in their homes. Although this practice of 'domiciliary' nursing continued until the start of the Second World War there was a fall in demand. Now that the voluntary hospitals were highly regarded, many wealthy patients were choosing to be treated as in-patients. In this they were encouraged by their doctors, who preferred having access to the improved facilities available in the larger hospitals for which they could charge accordingly. Class barriers, for patients if not the institutions, had been irrevocably breached during the First World War with wounded or sick officers recognising and appreciating the benefits of the professional nursing care and treatment they had received in military hospitals. Post-war, as the wealthy turned to hospitals for treatment in increasing numbers, there was an expansion in the building of private patients' blocks attached to the larger, more prestigious hospitals to cater for their comfort and privacy. These wealthy patients contributed to both the building funds and, by the fees charged, to the maintenance of these facilities and to the medical and nursing costs.

Private nursing homes also flourished to meet the new demand but the nurses working in them were largely untrained. This was of great concern, particularly to the College of Nursing. In 1927 the College of Nursing had urged the government to support their proposal that all nurses working in nursing homes should be registered. However, the Select Committee on Nursing Homes took the view that only the nurse in charge of the home needed to be registered. In the mid-1920s the College also presented a Bill to Parliament demanding the registration and inspection of nursing homes. Doctors, who gained substantially from fees of patients in these homes, did not welcome government interference and therefore did not support the College's petition. However, the Society of Medical Officers of Health did support the Bill, which was passed as the Registration of Nursing Homes Act in 1927. For the College of Nursing it was a matter of great pride: they had made a good case for the safeguarding of public health and the maintenance of standards of nursing against strong opposition from the BMA, and they had won.

Regrettably, petty squabbling, unseemly in-fighting and rampant snobbery had marred progress in College committees in the period leading up to registration. After the 1919 Registration of Nurses Act had been passed, Ethel Fenwick, a self-professed champion of 'liberty and self-government', remained a dominant and at times a somewhat negative force in proceedings, determined to keep professional nursing the exclusive domain of upper class women like herself. She and her followers sought every way possible to keep the matrons of the Poor Law hospitals, and the nurses they represented whom they regarded as poorly trained and ignorant, out of the decision-making process.

In the early twentieth century the Poor Law infirmaries began to employ more qualified nurses and probationers. Between 1901 and 1937 the numbers of paid staff in these hospitals increased eight-fold, by far eclipsing the rate of growth in nursing staff in the voluntary hospitals. One significant factor was the need to remove pauper nurses (often recruited from recovering workhouse inmates) from the wards and replace them with probationers. As a consequence of the 1929 Local Government Act the responsibility for administering Poor Law infirmaries was transferred from the Poor Law Guardians to local government authorities such as town councils, where they became the responsibility of the Medical Officer of Health, and increasingly re-branded as municipal general hospitals, like the former isolation hospitals. Over the next ten years the rates of pay offered to nurses and probationers rose, the hours of work reduced and accommodation improved, making municipal hospitals much more attractive to work in, and further compounding the difficulties faced by the voluntary hospitals. In an attempt to increase staffing levels, some voluntary hospitals even reduced the age of entry for their training schools from twenty-one to nineteen.

However, with the increasing numbers of probationers now working on wards the GNC was keen to maintain high standards in training and prevent these young girls from being used as merely another pair of hands with little hope of being equipped to pass the State final examinations. The Council's drive to raise standards of training and 'approve' hospital training schools proved ineffective without paid inspectors to monitor progress, given that hospitals did not have the funds to invest in the facilities to meet the high standards it demanded. A syllabus for training was introduced in the early 1920s and in 1925 the first national examinations were held but there was a failure rate of 40 per cent. The high failure rate continued for several years and was a cause for concern. In response, in 1937 the College introduced an entrance examination for probationers to try to ensure that candidates had an acceptable level of education necessary to undertake the training. It was not until after the Second World War, over twenty years after registration had started, that the GNC could finally employ paid inspectors to supervise and monitor the standards within training schools.

The registration of nurses was closely tied to wider developments in the professionalisation of nursing and improving standards of medical care. The trained nurse was now judged by whether or not she was registered. Nurses who were registered stood a much better chance of being employed than those who were not. Moreover, those trained as general nurses were seen as having reached 'the top'. Increasingly, general nurses perceived that also gaining at least the first part of the midwifery qualification would make them unassailable in terms of employability. The conditions of service for nurses thus varied widely as did the quality of nursing.

Enrolled nurses and the second tier of training

The increasing demand for registered nurses meant that only those institutions that paid well and offered good conditions of service attracted them, leaving the unqualified and unregistered nurses to fill in the gaps elsewhere. Registration had highlighted the deficiencies in nurse provision: there were simply not enough women engaging in nursing as a career. While the work of the GNC undoubtedly raised standards for trained nurses across the country, by setting the bar so high it put off many who might otherwise have been attracted to nursing. For women in the inter-war years there was now a wide range of occupations open to them. Nursing, with its restrictive life-style and vocational commitment, had to compete with retail and office work as well as the emergence of new careers allied to the vast welfare sector, such as social work. In 1937 the Athlone Committee was set up to look into ways in which nursing recruitment and retention could be improved. Among many recommendations, the creation of a second tier of trained nurses, mainly for those currently working as assistant nurses, was proposed. There was, however, little enthusiasm for this proposal at the time.

Impact on district nurses

From the introduction of nurse registration in 1919, district nurses were disadvantaged. Their training, since the turn of the century, had included six months of midwifery and six months working with the sick poor in their homes. It meant that many district nurses were not equipped to pass the examination set by the GNC. However, the Queen's Institute (founded in 1889 as the Queen Victoria Jubilee Institute for Nurses) supported trained nurses whose role as 'Queen's Nurses' steadily developed and, over time, the village nurses and midwives were supervised by Queen's Nurses which helped to bring uniformity and improved standards to their training and work.

District nursing responded to the changing roles of women in society and in 1917 for the first time salaried, as opposed to voluntary, superintendents were employed in district nursing training homes. During the First World War there was a slight decline in the numbers of district nurses working nationally and this took time to recover post-war. The district nursing services along with the voluntary hospitals faced acute financial strain in the 1920s due to lack of donations. But following registration, increasing numbers of nurses were attracted to district work, although this exacerbated the shortage of registered nurses in hospitals. A former Liverpool district nurse, Winifred Froom, provided a picture of the life of a rural district nurse in the early 1950s. In an interview given to Dr Patricia Starkey in the mid-1990s she recalled:

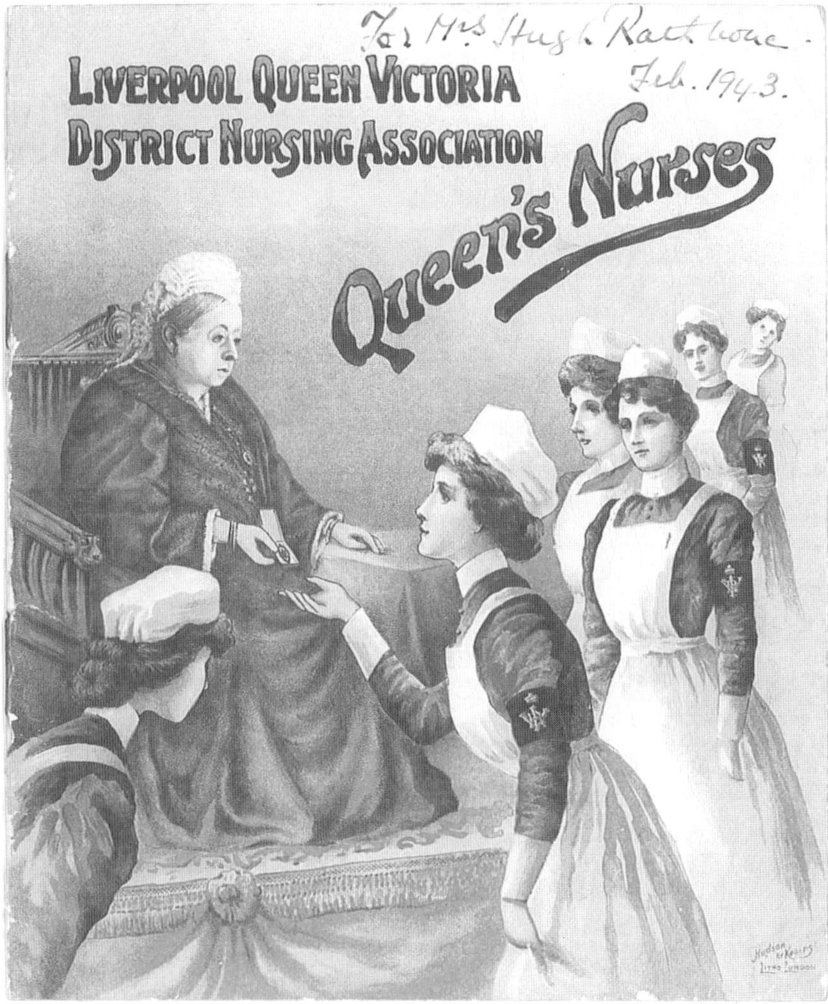

Figure 3.2 *front cover of Liverpool Queen Victoria District Nursing Association's booklet (Liverpool Record Office ref RAT610)*

> *In the homely parlours, or in the bedrooms, we conducted much the same kind of work as on the city rounds; dressings, bed baths, and of course a maternity case... there was the same anticipation of our arrival, but the difference lay in the greater responsibility borne by the nurse, alone in her cottage, with only the telephone to link her with the doctor or the nearest hospital.*

With increasing numbers of the public choosing to use hospitals during the inter-war years – from both the lower and upper sectors of society – there was consequently a decline in the demand for the district nurse. Traditionally their work had been with the sick poor and chronic sick at home and with the changes in public perception of health services in general, their role began to change. One way in which this happened was the need for careful monitoring of new drug therapies and wound treatments once patients were discharged from hospital care.

Fever nursing

Another significant branch of nursing that had developed during the late nineteenth and early twentieth century was fever nursing. Although the devastating epidemics of cholera and smallpox were no longer regular events in Liverpool, there were still plenty of infectious diseases, such as diphtheria, scarlet fever, and tuberculosis that required specialised medical and nursing care. Liverpool had founded a Fever Hospital in 1801. By the 1870s the town council was obliged to provide free isolation hospital accommodation for infectious diseases patients (and they were required by law to be compulsorily isolated – difficult to achieve in most homes). Netherfield Hospital was established and expanded to meet this requirement. In 1901 Liverpool council decided it needed further isolation accommodation, preferably outside the city to reduce the risk of disease transmission, so it bought a large plot of land in the then rural area of Fazakerley. The Annexe Hospital opened there, providing 160 fever beds. In 1906 it was expanded to 510 beds and renamed as the City Hospital Fazakerley. Tuberculosis patients were given a dedicated sanatorium there in 1920 with 245 beds.

Margaret Smith did her fever nurse training at Fazakerley, beginning in 1945, aged 17:

> *Fever nursing treatment consisted of good basic general nursing, hygiene and medication. Junior nursing tasks included bed-making, bedpan rounds, bed bathing, feeding (babies and adults), ward cleanliness (damp dusting) and tidiness, the preparation of dressings and packing them in drums for autoclaving; boiling up used glass syringes in the steriliser. Dealing with soiled linen and sterilising bed pans made the junior 'Queen of the sluice and linen cupboard'.*
>
> *The hours of work were from 8am to 8pm, with two hours off duty, with one and a half days off per week. All members of staff were resident in Nurses' Homes. Juniors slept in 4-bed dormitory rooms. There were*

communal bathrooms and toilets –and no heating. Lectures had to be attended either on-duty or off-duty or even on nights off. During all this time there was learning from senior colleagues on the ward.

Working on cubicle wards required great care to avoid cross-infection. Gowns had to be worn on entry to the cubicle, scrubbing hands and arms up to the elbows with Lysol solution before leaving. Sulphonamides were the main drug treatment until Penicillin, which was introduced during my training... For diphtheria cases when necessary a steam tent was put together with a sheet draped over a screen – a beautiful copper steam kettle stood on a stool, positioned with the spout near the patient. Failing this treatment a tracheotomy was necessary – on a table on the ward, the prepared pack opened and, with a good light available, in minutes the gasping was relieved.

On the open wards there were fires in the centre of the ward and these were kept stoked up by the junior on night duty. A junior on night duty spent the whole 12 hours on the ward. A light meal was delivered by the porter. Drinks and refreshments were taken when time allowed. The night sister visited twice nightly – travelling sometimes by bicycle! We were always busy, non-stop working, but very happy days. No regrets.

The origins of the NHS

Health care in Britain before 5 July 1948 was dependent on the wealth of the individual. The state had progressively taken on responsibility for some aspects of health, especially public health, and the health of those deemed worthy of welfare support. One can date this back to the Victorian Poor Law and to the sanitary reforms that initiated compulsory vaccination schemes and disease surveillance. It was partly the pressure of the newly enfranchised working class men after 1867 that prompted the existing political parties – the Liberals and the Conservatives – to respond to concerns about ill-health (now firmly associated with poverty since the work of Engels and Chadwick), and to offer a more robust state health security net.

This took shape under the reforming Liberal government between 1906 and 1911, which saw the institution of school medical inspections, infant and maternal welfare clinics, and a National Health Insurance scheme. Panel Doctors were appointed from independent general practitioners (GPs) who owned their own practices. They received a capitation fee from the government for providing basic health care to the working men who had paid the compulsory contribution to the scheme. Most men also continued to pay into the private health insurance and friendly society schemes which covered their wives and children, and who were cared for by the same GPs. A Ministry of Health was established in 1919, which helped to institutionalise the philosophy that certain health issues were the natural responsibility of the state. Yet this steady expansion of state-funded health services, which required medical staffing, did not sit well with the medical profession. For many, it was a 'thin end of the wedge' attack on their freedom from control and ability to determine their own incomes.

Although there had been discussion of going further than the Liberal welfare reforms, the inter-war period saw little change. There had been an innovative report prepared by Lord Dawson in 1920 for the Minister of Health's Consultative Council on Medical and Allied Services, in which he used his military expertise to propose a reorganisation of Britain's diverse health care providers into regional hierarchies of primary and secondary facilities (primary being general practice, and secondary referring to hospitals and specialist treatments – the first time these terms were applied to British health care). The general proposal – that 'the best means of maintaining health and cutting disease should be made available to all citizens' was backed up by the report of the Royal Commission on National Health Insurance in 1928, which suggested 'divorcing the medical service entirely from the insurance system and recognising it along with all other public health activities as a service to be supported from the general public funds'. This would have forced the pace on greater collaboration between the state's health care services (mainly municipal hospitals and clinics – some of them former Poor Law institutions) and those provided for the majority of the population through private general practitioners and voluntary (independent) hospitals.

By the mid-1930s many of the voluntary hospitals were experiencing financial crises. Their income could not keep pace with the costs of medical treatment. In 1891 some 88 per cent of their income had come from gifts and investments; by 1938 this had reduced to 35 per cent and patients now contributed 59 per cent of voluntary hospital income either out of their own pockets or through insurance schemes. It left these hospitals vulnerable to economic conditions. Of the 145 voluntary hospitals in London in 1932, 60 failed to balance their books, and by 1938 these hospitals were pleading with the government for state support. The plaintive cry: 'funds urgently needed: beds closed' suggested to many people that the voluntary hospital sector might not be worth saving.

Other proposals were emerging, which reflected their authors' primary concerns. The British Medical Association in 1930 had proposed extending the insurance coverage to the whole population and a coordinated regional hospital service. The Socialist Medical Association (SMA) in 1933 proposed a more radical solution – that all healthcare should be provided free at the point of use through one scheme, funded either by taxation or national insurance, and administered by local government. This was adopted as official Labour Party policy in 1934. In 1937 the *Report on the British Health Services* by the think tank PEP (Political and Economic Planning) proposed similar nationalised services, to extend primary health care from the 43 per cent who were currently covered by Panel doctors under NHI to the whole population. This would also have suited many GPs who were not well off, and who supplemented their panel work with sessions in hospitals and occupational health services.

Catalysts for change

From 1938 senior civil servants within the Ministry of Health began to hold discussions on the future of the health services. The threat of another war, however, forced the government to suspend its planning. It temporarily commandeered all hospitals to form an Emergency Medical Service (EMS), to provide free medical care for certain groups, and to fund the voluntary hospitals. As the war progressed its remit was extended to cover the majority of British people.

An Emergency Nursing Committee was created to work closely with the College of Nursing, the British Red Cross and the Order of St John of Jerusalem. This committee was charged with the task of preparing a register of those with any nursing experience, including assistants and auxiliary nurses. While thousands registered and were available to be employed by local authorities to fill the gaps left by qualified nurses required by the Armed Forces, many were married women and mothers needing to work part-time and locally and who therefore could not be posted to other areas. In establishing the Civil Nursing Reserve (CNR) the committee had hoped to avoid the problems created for the nursing profession by the VAD scheme a generation earlier and members of the Reserve were allocated in a variety of ways: in hospitals, First Aid posts, district nursing and on evacuation trains.

In Liverpool in 1938 Keith Monsarrat, a newly-retired surgeon at the David Lewis Northern Hospital, was appointed as Director of the

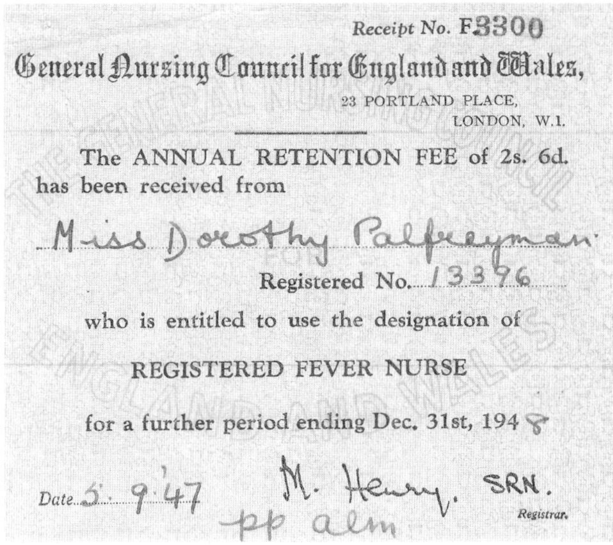
Receipt No. F3300

General Nursing Council for England and Wales,

23 PORTLAND PLACE,
LONDON, W.1.

The ANNUAL RETENTION FEE of 2s. 6d. has been received from

Miss Dorothy Palfreyman

Registered No. 13396

who is entitled to use the designation of

REGISTERED FEVER NURSE

for a further period ending Dec. 31st, 1948

Date 5. 9. 47 M. Henry. SRN. pp alm

Registrar.

Figure 3.3 *Dorothy Haig's (nee Palfreyman) Fever Nurse Registration receipt*

Emergency Hospital Scheme which was part of the EMS. He was, according to retired Liverpool surgeon, James Carmichael, a remarkable man, *'a territorial [army officer], and was both a good doctor and a good organiser – a rare combination…'*. From an office based at the Liverpool Medical Institution at the top of Mount Pleasant, Monsarrat had the power to requisition beds, move hospitals and decide who would and would not, be called up or designated as in a 'reserved' occupation. In 1939 there were nearly 50 hospitals across Merseyside, providing together over 9,000 beds. These were split between the four teaching hospitals with almost 1,000 beds (the Royal, Northern, Southern and Stanley); the much larger municipal hospitals (Fazakerley, Walton, Mill Road and Smithdown Road) had over 2,600 beds, and in addition Belmont Road Hospital had up to 1,000 'chronic' beds.

The port of Liverpool was expected to be a target for aerial bombing. During the course of the war it handled almost 50 per cent of the imports into the country, including vast amounts of military equipment from the USA. It was clear that both the David Lewis Northern and the Royal Southern Hospitals, sited close to the docks, were vulnerable to the risk of bombing. Most of the beds had to be relocated leaving only outpatients and casualty departments open. Within a couple of weeks the Royal Southern was relocated to Fazakerley Infectious Diseases' Hospital, and the David Lewis Northern took over St Katherine's Teacher Training College in Childwall. To cope with the anticipated heavy casualties from bombing, half the patients of Highfield

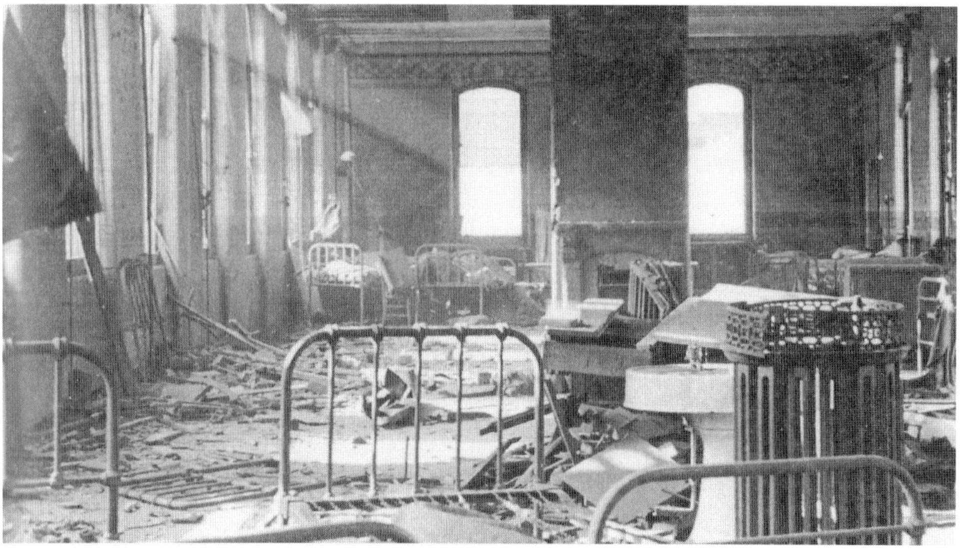

Figure 3.4 *Bomb damage on Ward 8 at the Liverpool Royal Infirmary*

Tuberculosis Sanatorium were discharged freeing up a further 200 beds. Mill Road Hospital with its 700 beds in West Derby was designated a casualty hospital though it also continued to be a maternity hospital. Dorothy Haig had begun her fever nursing course at Fazakerley in 1940, aged 18. Her experiences were common to most student nurses in wartime, with hugely increased responsibilities:

> *There were searchlights and a mobile gun in the grounds. When the sirens went all the counterpanes were removed and used as shelter: mattress and child placed under the bed and the base covered with a counterpane. At the sound of the 'All Clear' they went back to bed… In the Annexe, the old 'wooden' wards were occupied by servicemen. I nursed one ward full of servicemen with Scarlet Fever, on my own.*

Liverpool suffered sustained and increasingly devastating aerial bombardment between August 1940 and May 1941. In December 1940, Mill Road's Nurses' Home was hit. Student nurse Winifred Froom, who was in her second year of training at the hospital, recalled air-raid preparations:

> *Deep shelters had been dug outside the Nurses' Home. We were instructed to report to them unless on night duty. Some of the nurses refrained from*

going into the shelters, until someone in authority rounded them up, which was just as well, for when least expected, just before Christmas, the Nurses' Home received a stray bomb which sliced it in two. Luckily nobody was injured...

However in May 1941, during eight relentless days of bombing, once again Mill Road Hospital, thought to have been in a safe location away from the River Mersey and the docks, took a direct hit that destroyed a large part of the building including a maternity ward, killing mothers and babies as well as two midwives. Elsewhere in Mill Road hospital patients and medical staff were killed, including two medical students and two nurses in the operating theatre. The Royal also took a direct hit. It was a small bomb and although there was damage to the building there was no loss of life.

Pauline Derbin had started her nurse training in 1939 at Alder Hey. She was working at Garston during the Liverpool blitz of 1941:

Myself and a friend sneaked out in the evening to buy fish and chips. On the way back the bombers came over Liverpool. We sheltered under an army jeep eating our fish and chips and watched the 'fireworks'...

Dilys Greenhalgh started her training at Alder Hey Hospital during the war.

The nurses' home at Alder Hey was huge, three stories high with old lifts, the corridors were heated but there was no heating in the rooms so sometimes we slept two in a single bed so we could have two blankets instead of one... I remember the hospital ships landing in Liverpool with injured forces and all nurses second year and above had to go on duty to help... dozens of military ambulances travelled up Prescot Road as far as you could see.

Mill Road beds were moved to Highfield Sanatorium where six more TB wards had to be cleared to make way for over 300 acute beds. Although these beds were urgently needed, the early discharge of TB patients put their families at much greater risk with a consequent rise in numbers diagnosed by the end of the war. The 'new' hospital was renamed Broadgreen where, eventually with the addition of hutted wards, there were over 750 beds.

The large numbers of assistants and auxiliaries employed during the war under the Civil Nursing Reserve scheme had no recognised standard of training. This eventually gave the Ministry of Health a valid reason to resolve the contentious issue of a second tier of trained nurses first mooted around 1905 and later, in 1937, proposed by the Athlone Committee. The 1943 Nurses Act gave assistant nurses the opportunity to undertake a less academically onerous statutory training over two years. On successful completion of state examinations these nurses were to be entered on the 'roll' held by the GNC becoming State Enrolled nurses within the profession.

Partly as a publicity exercise to lift war-time spirits in the depths of the Blitz, the national coalition government commissioned a Liberal academic and civil servant William Beveridge to produce a report on the potential for post-war welfare reform. Beveridge went further than his brief allowed, and his 1942 report, *On Social Security and Allied Services*, was an instant public hit – selling over 600,000 copies – unheard of for a dry government publication. The Treasury, however, were dismayed by the cost implications. They had thought he was engaged to tidy up the existing administration, rather than to propose such a radical new policy. What Beveridge had produced was a blueprint for tackling what he called the 'five giant evils' that currently damaged Britain: squalor, ignorance, want, idleness and disease. The state's responsibility for the welfare of its citizens should be 'from cradle to grave'. For health he proposed a comprehensive service, 'without a charge on treatment at any point'.

The Conservatives, led by Winston Churchill, the coalition government's Prime Minister, had been unhappy to be pushed into action by Beveridge's audacious report, but they had no choice but to allow a series of White Papers to be produced. The one proposing a National Health Service was prepared in 1944. Unexpectedly, it proposed central rather than local government management, as well as the fundamental principle of free treatment for all. The issue of how to integrate GPs into a national system was equally challenging. The White Paper acknowledged that a more equitable distribution of GPs was required, but the medical profession was clear that they wished to remain free from any sort of state control. Nobody was entirely happy with the 1944 White Paper, but, crucially, no party felt totally alienated by it.

At the end of the Second World War the National Government was dissolved, and at the May 1945 general election the Labour party won an unexpected landslide victory. The new Minister of Health was a Welshman, Aneurin – known as Nye – Bevan (1897-1960). A 45 year-old Welsh former miner, he was one of Labour's most charismatic and visionary politicians. His new proposals went much further than any of the interwar discussions or Beveridge's proposals. He wanted a national

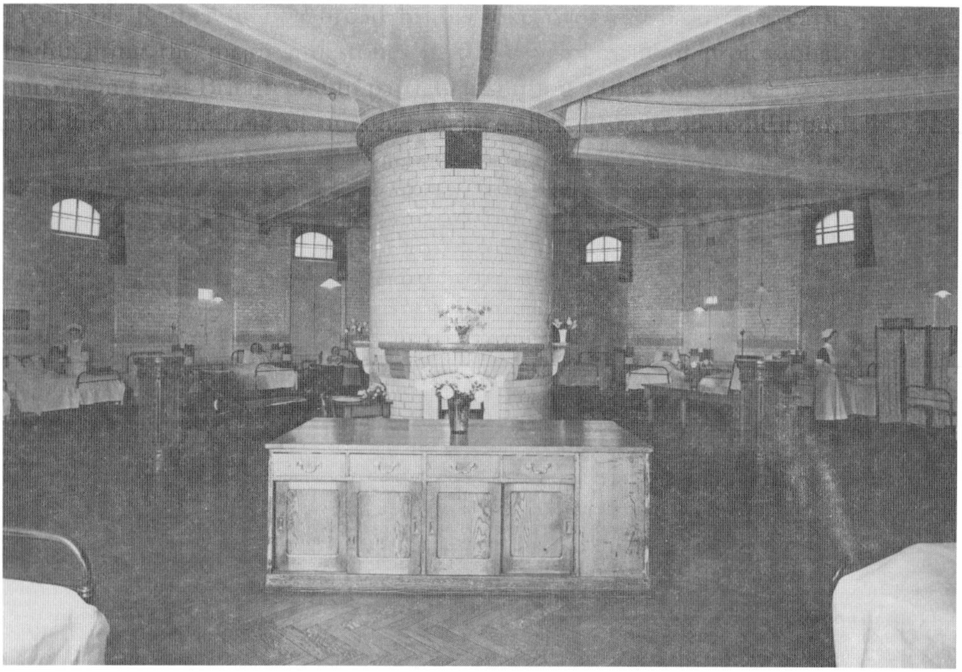

Figure 3.5 *Blackout: bricked up windows in one of the Royal Infirmary's circular wards, 1943*

takeover of all hospitals, a health service to be available to all without charge, the end to selling GP practices, and funding to be primarily by central taxation, with only a small contribution from National Insurance. The key principle enshrined in the March 1946 Bill was that health was a right, not a commodity to be bought or sold, or subject to market forces.

After many months of negotiation on issues of finance, structure and management, the 1946 NHS Act was passed. It was essentially a compromise, and one which set up fundamental structural weaknesses, especially by divorcing medical care (hospitals and some GP work) from health care (local authorities and some GP work). The British Medical Association, with the popular radio doctor Charles Hill as its articulate spokesman, therefore initially opposed the NHS Act, fearing that it would be too intrusive on professional freedom, and turn all healthcare into a local government service. At the first vote its members rejected it. After some last minute negotiations, Bevan got the commitments from the medical profession that he needed. He was later to recall, in his most famous quote, that he had 'stuffed their mouths with gold'. The NHS was therefore born, on its due date, 5 July 1948. Bevan commented on the scale of his achievement: 'This is the biggest single experiment in social services that the world has ever seen undertaken'.

The public reaction was one of overwhelming relief. For the working classes the threat of doctors' and hospital bills had been a chronic concern. Now there were no more bills (unless of course the patient opted to jump the NHS queue and pay for private treatment). Although many of the nationalised hospitals were not fit for purpose, there was at least now a government commitment to a more equitable allocation of resources between regions. And the new regional health authorities, with their mandate to plan services for populations which ranged from one to five million, were able to develop effective data collection systems, and provide specialist services. It was an extraordinarily efficient system, and from its outset the focus of international envy. But it was now the government that worried about the bills, and they had good cause, despite the inherent logic of this part-integrated system. During planning in 1945, the estimate for the annual cost of the NHS had been £170 million. In its first full year of operation – 1949 – it cost £305 million.

While the public may have been relieved at the reality of 'free' healthcare those unfortunate enough to have to be admitted to hospitals in the late 1940s must have been concerned at the lack of nurses on the wards. The 1946 NHS Act did not consider the issue of nurse education or the administration to run it. There was a critical shortage of trained nurses and fear among those working that under the new system they would be moved about to other hospitals to fill gaps rather like military service personnel were. Both working and living conditions in hospitals had over the years deteriorated dramatically and qualified nurses were leaving the profession in droves. Not only were they discontent with the lowering of standards and shortages of trained staff during and after the war, there were other factors contributing to this exodus from the profession. Women had more choices in employment but crucially there were also fewer of them to make those choices. Between 1931 and 1951 the numbers of single women in Britain declined. Nursing was in transition, hospitals had for too long regarded student nurses as cheap labour and things had to change. There was much work to be done to get the profession on to a strong footing for the challenges of the new Health Service.

Daphne Cunningham trained at the Liverpool Royal Infirmary between 1944 and 1948, and witnessed the transformation of the hospital from war-time conditions into the NHS:

I had been put off applying to London because of the doodlebug raids. I remember as a junior nurse lighting fires on the wards, and cleaning beside lockers each evening particularly fluff from the castors, polishing the brass knob and rail, putting everything away inside leaving just a tray cloth on the top (put there to muffle sound and not disturb patients sleeping). There were no curtains around beds, we had to lug wooden screens to the bed for privacy. There were no windows at the Royal, it was really grim they had all been bricked up though we did have electric lights over the head of each bed. In 1946, half way through my training, we had workmen hammering every day putting the windows back in all over the hospital.

There were the 'shawlies', three women side by side on hands and knees, who scrubbed and scrubbed the long corridors from one end to the other every day, lots of chat and banter, they were always cheerful... Hospital staff returned to the wards following war service... it set aside three 32-bed wards each with an extra 8 beds added, for wounded soldiers. Nobody had requisitioned additional tea mugs, so we had to re-use mugs from those served first... There were white counterpanes with a circle woven into the fabric in the centre with the words 'Liverpool Royal Infirmary' around a Liver bird which had to lie in the centre of the bed the right way up... I remember Sister Whitley-Jones, known as the 'bomber' (after the Armstrong Whitworth Whitley aircraft, a World War Two bomber), in charge of the orthopaedic ward – very efficient but a stickler for dust, prone to be rather sarcastic, as many of the sisters were...

Unlike at the end of the First World War when there had been a surplus of women volunteering to work as nurses in hospitals up and down the country, in 1939 there was a dearth of both trained nurses and those wanting to start training. The creation of the Civil Nursing Service had not attracted the anticipated large numbers of women to the wards. The situation was so serious that at the end of the war over 30,000 beds were closed across the country due to the shortage of nursing staff. The reasons for this were complex: girls were now educated to secondary level which greatly contributed to the expansion of opportunities for employment for young women. Another factor was the lowering of both the age at which training could commence and a lowering of the standard required to apply, to combat the falling numbers coming into nursing in the 1930s, which had a detrimental affect on morale within hospitals. This was part of the backdrop to the beginning of Britain's new National Health Service in 1948.

Chapter 4

Nursing and the National Health Service

FROM AS EARLY AS 1931 discussions were being held about the amalgamation of the four main teaching hospitals in Liverpool: the Liverpool Royal Infirmary, the David Lewis Northern, the Royal Southern and the Liverpool Stanley hospitals. This idea came from the University of Liverpool who wanted the Liverpool Royal Infirmary to become the University Clinic, a centre for teaching and research. The outcome was the creation of a Voluntary Hospital Board to oversee future discussions and planning and in 1934 the idea of amalgamation was approved in principle by the Associated Voluntary Hospital Board. Momentum slowly built up, and a conference held in 1936 for representatives of the main teaching hospitals led to the Liverpool United Hospitals Act in July 1937. The impending war interfered with Liverpool's hospital amalgamation plans, but there was greater collaboration between the hospitals, now known as the Liverpool United Hospitals Group, for the training and provision of nursing staff. Applications for training were made to the hospital group, and probationers were allocated their hospital placements rather than applying to a specific hospital. Classroom training continued to be delivered in the building originally provided by Rathbone in 1862, adjacent to the Liverpool Royal Infirmary.

In the post-war years student nurses were still expected to live-in at the nurses' homes attached to each of the main hospitals. The Royal Infirmary had started building a new nurses' home during the 1920s on land on the corner of Ashton Street and Prescot Street. Though called Cedar House it was universally known as the 'New Home'. It was

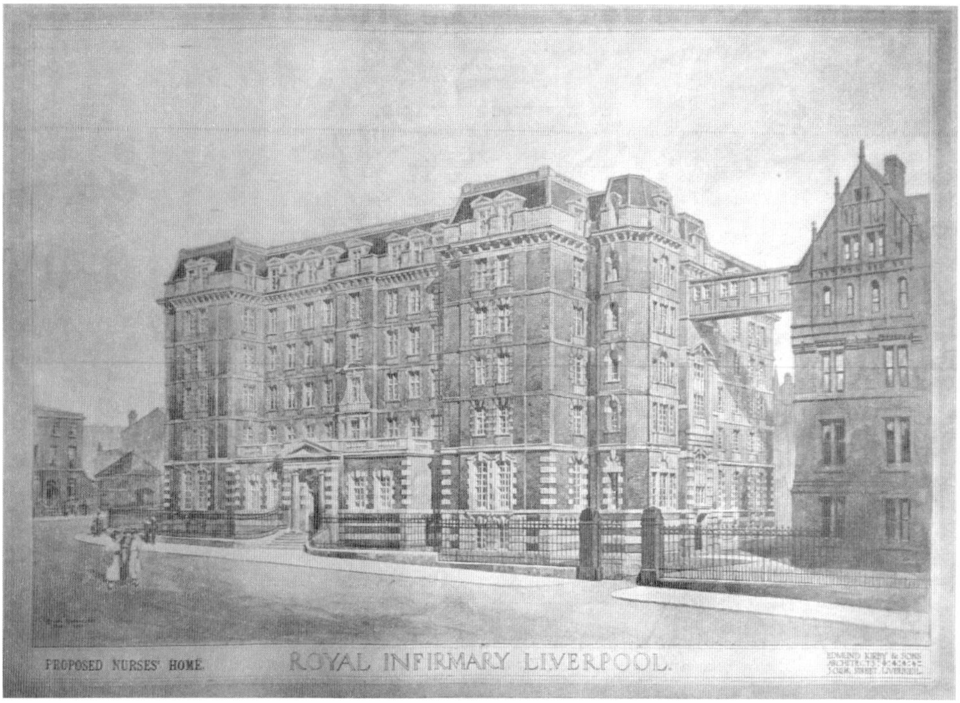

Figure 4.1 *Architect's drawing of Cedar House, the New Nurses' Home at the Royal Infirmary, 1931 (courtesy of the Beresford collection, Royal Liverpool and Broadgreen University Hospital Trust archives)*

finally completed by 1933 and it provided more spacious and modern accommodation for the nursing staff.

Life was strictly controlled with a Home Sister in charge of most aspects of their lives. The front door was locked by 10.30pm. In 1954 a new Preliminary Training School (or PTS as it was known) for students of the constituent schools of nursing of the United Liverpool Hospital was opened at Woolton Manor for the initial classroom instruction in the rudiments of nursing care. For the first eight weeks of training students lived there and had lessons. At the end of PTS students then moved in to the nurses' home at the hospital to which they were allocated. In the 1970s the rules were relaxed and while nurses were encouraged to live-in it was no longer compulsory. In 1978 the new Hospital College opened, as the first part of the new Royal Liverpool Hospital, and teaching was moved there from Woolton Manor.

The Cunningham twins (Elizabeth Mawdsley and Alison Rostance) trained at the Royal between 1957 and 1961, where their cousin Daphne Cunningham was senior sister on the tropical ward when they started their training:

> Elizabeth: *It was very special to be called a Royal nurse. I worked there, the ENT [Ear, Nose and Throat] hospital, Myrtle Street and Heswall Children's Hospital. We all had to live-in at the new home on the corner of Ashton Street unless we were on nights when we moved into the Old Home. There were also rooms for a time at No. 13 Rodney Street… Sister Addison was Home Sister. She was very strict, doors were locked [at 10.30 p.m.]… Daphne sometimes gave us a key so we could come in late, On our first ward most of the day was spent in the sluice, we were the lowest of the low.*

> Alison: *I always wanted to nurse and I loved it. I was very proud to be training at the Royal, so many eminent doctors, world-renowned, Professor Jeffcoate, Lord Cohen, Professor Clark. On our first day in Preliminary Training School (or PTS as it was universally known) we put on our yellow dresses, [we were] known as 'daffodils', really hideous, and were called 'Nurse' from then on. There was much giggling. Sister Laura Jones the senior tutor, was very good. We were told that we must never wear make-up as "it would make the patient feel disadvantaged". First year students were on duty by 7.30 – report, jobs, to sluices and sterilising room, all had to be spick and span… making 32 beds in half an hour by the clock! Then breakfasts, and wiping down every locker – there was lots of cleaning. All beds were pulled away from wall on one side, the cleaners did the floors, then the beds went back and then repeated the other side. Floors were mopped, and polished weekly. We used tea leaves to collect the dust. We were never allowed to sit down while on duty. We always stood to attend to patients, feeding etc…*

> Elizabeth: *There were different collars to denote year of training – first year the same colour as the dress, 2nd year Peter Pan detachable collar and 3rd year it was like a dog collar.*

> Alison: *When you passed your State [exam] you went into 'frillies' – starched cap, it was a nightmare to starch and fold correctly… everyone clapped on the ward when you appeared in it.*

> Elizabeth: *We couldn't afford to go out much. We went home to Birkenhead on days off. Later on we sometimes went to dances or to clubs like*

The Cabin, there was another called The Catacombs... once a year there was a most fantastic hospital Ball.

Alison: *In our third year, on the day of the Ball I was on a split duty. I had my hair done in the afternoon break, backcombed very high. When I went back on duty I could only perch my cap and clip it on the top. Sister said, 'And who do you think you are, Alice in Wonderland?' She pulled me into the office, yanked off my cap and squashed all my hair in underneath it. We still had fun at the Ball though.*

Eunice Trotman also trained at the Royal between 1959 and 1963:

We had to do three months night duty a year, ten 12-hour nights on, four off, a killer. I remember the ward report round the ward desk, the night nurse read out the report. The first year you worked so hard but felt fortunate to be at the Royal. There was a brilliant Orthopaedic sister, the "bomber", Sister Whitley-Jones. She was very fierce but a brilliant nurse, and everyone knew and respected her. In my PTS there were only about sixteen of us. Ten finished training so there was a lot of wastage.

In 1960, following the 1957 Nurses Act, which abolished the supplementary nursing registers and created a single register divided into parts, the Royal College of Nursing (RCN) relaxed many of its recruitment restrictions. In particular, it encouraged more men to enter the profession, especially into mental nursing. This was also a response to the increasing shortages of trained nurses, which prompted the Minister of Health, Enoch Powell, to look for temporary nursing immigrants from Commonwealth countries. The Platt Committee also recommended some changes to nurse education when it reported in 1964, but there was still lack of vision on the bigger organisational issues, such as the use of 'nursing auxiliaries' – the untrained women who provided increasingly large amounts of patient care in the post-war period, much to the annoyance of the RCN.

Alongside this, Powell's radical plans to modernise District General Hospitals prompted a wider review of nursing, which was published as the Salmon Report in 1966. This introduced managerial grades above ward sister to replace the traditional hospital matron. This however was criticised for taking senior nurses away from the bedside, and hindering the career development and clinical practice of the ward sister. The introduction of 'Functional Management' in the 1960s also disrupted nurses' roles. The new domestic supervisors now controlled aspects of ward life such as cleaning and laundry. Nurses were increasingly instructed not to undertake 'non-nursing' duties.

Each of the hospitals in the United Liverpool Hospital Group – the Royal, the David Lewis Northern, the Royal Southern, the Stanley and the Royal Liverpool Children's Hospitals – had formed its own Nurses League in the inter-war era, in common with hospitals around the country. These Leagues offered nurses the chance to stay in touch with other nurses trained at the same hospitals. They formed an extension to the 'family' of nurses, many of whom were fiercely loyal to their training institutions.

Jane Boag-Munroe, started her SRN training in 1969 at the United Liverpool Hospitals School of Nursing at Woolton Manor. She was the last president of the United Liverpool Hospital's Nurses League in the 1980s, (not to be confused with the Liverpool Royal Infirmary Nurses' League which still meets annually). Nurses have always valued their professional history, closely guarding the heritage and traditions laid down by their forebears. That is not to say that a little gentle irreverence does not also have its place in bringing together the old and the new. Boag-Munroe remembered some of the nurses from the Liverpool Branch of the Royal College of Nursing washing the memorial to Florence Nightingale which is on the garden wall of the original District Nurse Training School at the corner of Princes Avenue and Parliament Street. 'Giving Flo a Bath!' was a publicity event for Nurses' Day.

Those applying to train in Liverpool came from far and wide including the Isle of Man, Scotland and Ireland. The Royal had a long tradition of training Welsh girls, as well as local girls and many from the south of England, whereas at Sefton General, Broadgreen and Walton and the other former municipal hospitals they had a much broader mix of local girls, some boys, mature students as well as those from Wales, Scotland, Ireland and other nationalities.

Christine Hughes started her SRN course at the Royal in January 1963:

> *I remember Sister Laura Jones greeting us on first day at Woolton Manor for PTS. She was the main tutor – rather strict, as were all the staff in those days, some more than others. As we were only young girls then and most of us leaving home for the first time she tended to be rather like a mother hen, but she was always well-respected by all the girls and I look back on her with fondness. However, I don't think she enjoyed the Beatles music popular at that time which was played incessantly by one of the nurses.*

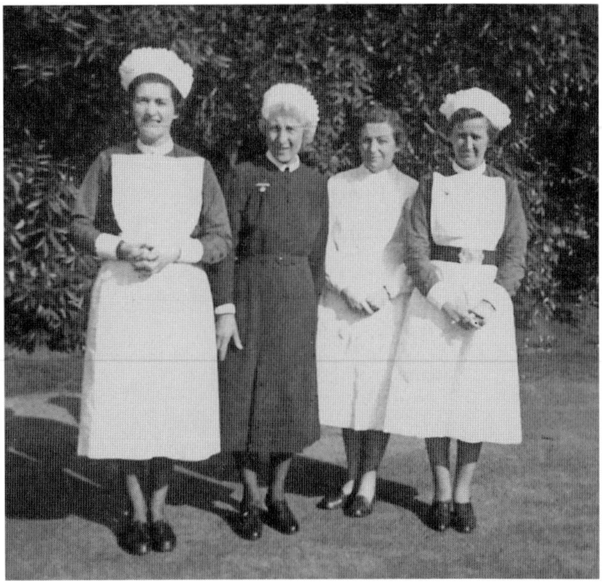

Figure 4.2 *Sister Laura Jones, Nurse Tutor (second left) with colleagues at Woolton Manor 1963 (photograph courtesy of Mrs C. Hughes)*

> *I can tell you there was one sister at the Royal, no names mentioned as she is still here, who terrified every young nurse she came into contact with. If she came one way we tried to disappear the other. However, the person I remember with the deepest respect and fondness is Sister Yule. She is the one person who was wonderful in every way to all she met. She was gentle and kind and although strict, all the nurses and patients loved her. They were happy times and sad times, we were just young girls but we had to grow up quickly. The friendships we shared helped us to get through. I had great admiration for Miss Rebecca Haynes, a tutor in a million. I would choose to go back and do exactly the same all over again.*

Claire Byrne started her SRN training at Whiston Hospital in 1970:

> *I was the only Irish girl in my PTS, I arrived from Ireland by ship early on Saturday 7 September 1970 and was collected and brought to Whiston, I was 18 years old and it was my first time away from home. Our bedrooms were at the end of a long corridor. The room had two single beds, a chest of drawers between them and a small wardrobe at the end of each bed. The rooms were so small that the wardrobe doors would only open half way… I made lifelong friends.*

Gillian Ormsby, commenced SRN training at the United Liverpool Hospitals in 1973:

We stayed at Woolton Manor but travelled on a coach to the School of Nursing. I worked at the Royal Southern Hospital, the LRI and Myrtle Street and Maternity hospitals... the old nurses' home at LRI was like a prison in design... The great experience and knowledge we gained, the support from clinical tutors and responsibility we had as students... some strict ward sisters, the neat and tidy beds... pillow cases facing the end of the ward!

Dame Lorna Muirhead DBE trained in Birmingham before moving to Liverpool to take up a midwifery post at the Liverpool Maternity Hospital in Oxford Street.

You either love or hate midwifery, I never wanted to go back to general. Liverpool Maternity Hospital in 1965 was a tremendous place with world "greats" like Professor Sir Norman Jeffcoate, Robert Minnitt who gave us gas and air, and Cyril Clarke who pioneered Rhesus research... I was 23, I could smell excellence and I knew I wanted to be part of it. I spent nearly 40 years working there and saw huge changes in the management of labour, the survival of women and the improvement in mortality and morbidity of babies... an amazing revolution.

One of the key developments that Muirhead witnessed was better pain control in labour:

Liverpool had one of the very first epidural services in country. At the time, in the mid-1960s in London, the rich and famous were talking about this wonderful epidural analgesia which they spent £100 a time having. At that time the women of Toxteth were having them free. But the point was that women really had choice about pain control, and for me that was a wonderful thing... that was very positive. If you have seen the [TV] series 'Call the Midwife' – that was my time – I was the girl on the bicycle, I was the girl who lived in a great big home, not with nuns but with other midwives, going out day and night delivering babies in pretty dire conditions.

Muirhead also commented on the post-war changing culture of nursing, which reflected broader advances in women's rights:

In 1965 when I wanted to be married I had to ask permission of the hospital. There were a very, very few people who were married and the workforce in the main was of single women. The other great leap forward

> *was that after I had my children and wanted to go back to work I needed to be part-time. This was an amazing departure and again it was before the Medical Board to see if I could, if it was right, to work part time. Now you look at the part-time workers in the Health Service, it's taken for granted. But it was a huge thing... The other big thing was the right of women to have a mortgage. Most of the sisters and nurses before that time lived in nurses' homes and viewed retirement with great difficulty because they not only lost their profession but they lost their homes as well.*

She has strong feelings too about the language of nursing, and the impact of the apprenticeship system and new management hierarchies on standards:

> *How dare we change me from a ward sister to a ward manager? What is special about 'manager'? There's something very special about a ward sister. And when you change language you start to change the meaning of things. So that's what we were, an identifiable workforce. And you put that starched apron on, you become something professional, the public like it, I think it's very, very important to have that identity.*
>
> *In the apprentice model one of the great advantages used to be because you started from the bottom, you soon got to know if you could deal with the sort of things that we dealt with. You know, making patients comfortable doing those sorts of things. This lack of hierarchical structures, lack of charge, I see very much in my work in professional misconduct at the Nurses and Midwives Council (NMC). Much of what I see there would have been dealt with in the olden days by the ward sister, in the sluice. Because people are going to make mistakes. It's not misconduct coming before us at the NMC – we see too many people who are themselves victims of organisational failure.*

There were other hospitals in Liverpool that were not eligible to join the United Liverpool Hospitals Group when it was established before the NHS, because they were funded by the local authority. These were the municipal hospitals – many of which like Walton and Mill Road, had started life in the nineteenth century as Poor Law infirmaries, and as such carried a social stigma which even lasted into the early years of the NHS. There were also municipal isolation hospitals such as Fazakerley (later renamed Aintree Hospital), and smaller institutions such as Sefton General Hospital. This was formerly known as the Smithdown Road Hospital and had originally been Toxteth Park Poor Law Workhouse. Following the start of the NHS in 1948, it changed its name for the final time to Sefton General Hospital. It closed in 2001 and was eventually demolished.

Angela Hogg, who started her SRN training aged 18 at Sefton General Hospital in 1963, provides a personal perspective on the perceived hierarchy of Liverpool's hospitals:

> *The nurses at Sefton and Walton physically worked so hard due to the enormous throughput of patients and the poor nurse-patient ratio when compared with the smaller numbers of patients and the much higher ratio of staff at the Royal, the David Lewis Northern or the Royal Southern hospitals, despite the significant demands that medical student teaching made upon their working environments. [At Sefton] we often had extra beds in the centre of surgical wards for those admitted overnight. It was sheer, hard, physical slog.*
>
> *To be fair to all my colleagues at Sefton they did their best and the care, within the restrictions imposed upon them, was absolutely superb – kindly, skilled and very caring. But when you saw the nursing practice of the Northern nurses, their nursing techniques and procedures reminded me of the requirements of nursing procedures laid down by the Queen's Institute, in terms of their finesse and precision. [Northern nurses] took the trouble to use things like 'nightingales' [capes] around a patient's shoulders to groom their hair. Not at Sefton! But they were also much more limited in terms of the [nursing] procedures undertaken at Sefton or Walton because we [at Sefton] didn't have the medical students on the wards, taking blood pressures etc – we nurses, and very junior nurses, did that. So, it was very, very different but still they [United Hospital nurses] did feel that they were in some way superior!*

There were a variety of training courses for nurses by the 1970s, which allowed early specialisation, or entry into the profession at a younger age. Pam Kent started the combined Registered Sick Children's Nurse and State Registered Nurse Combined course (RSCN/SRN) in September 1975 at the United Liverpool Hospitals Training School. Her first experience was on Ward 4, female medical – one of the 'round' wards at the Royal:

> *I was shocked at the naked bodies, bottoms and boobs of all shapes and sizes! I remember the smell of Imperial Leather soap and Yardley's lavender talc. The cleaners were in control! We arranged bed baths etc around their cleaning routine. There were several fire places on a central chimney and walls lined with Victorian tiles… the tiles in the outpatients' department*

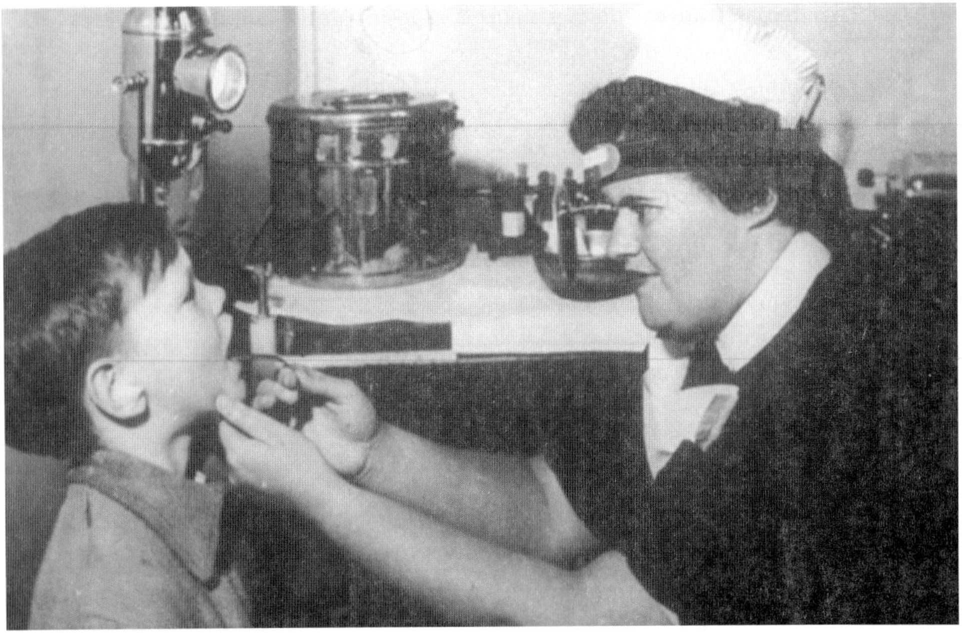

Figure 4.3 *Paediatric nurse with patient*

> *were particularly beautiful with green patterned pillars. At night the building was creepy. There was a short cut across the rooftops to the Nurses' Home which I once made wearing a red and white gingham bedpan gown covering my uniform. During my second year of training I was placed at Limekiln Lane Clinic with a health visitor. We visited from the cradle to the grave. We wore dresses of green cotton in summer and green crimplene in winter with a green felt hat! I remember visiting travelling families at a caravan site, and young and old families around Scotland Road. This was a revelation to me... a realisation that on the community I was able to see all the determinants of the patient's health rather than just a small snapshot in hospital. Health visiting seemed the ideal way to combine all aspects of my training.*

Cadet nurse courses were run in hospitals around Great Britain from the 1950s to 1970s. They catered for girls and boys who wanted to go on to train in nursing, allowing them to gain experience and a practical understanding from the age of 16. In the 1970s, despite having proved to be a successful route into nursing for many, the cadet nursing courses were stopped. However, in the late 1990s a modern cadet nursing course was established and has grown rapidly and successfully. Andrea

Spyropoulos, started as a cadet nurse at Sefton General Hospital in 1972 and commenced her SRN training in January 1973. As with so many of her colleagues, she shared an early vocation:

> *From being a young girl I always wanted to be a nurse... it absolutely changed my life because I came from a very poor background with very little opportunity. University was never, ever, ever an option for a kid like me, y'know. I grew up in Liverpool 5, in a large catholic area where the expectation for women was if you were lucky you got a secretarial job, so an education just wasn't discussed. When I told my mother I was going to go into nursing I think she thought that I just couldn't do it. But she was wrong... so it was a bit of a fight, but that desire to nurse set me on a pathway that exposed me to so many different things in terms of culture, academic achievement understanding people. At the time there was a big push for nurses, [but] for someone like me from a secondary modern school it was unusual to get into SRN training – they would try and push us into the enrolled nurse course, but I wouldn't be persuaded. I had the requirements you had to have 5 O-levels [for the SRN course] and I had them so I was going to apply.*
>
> *There was no choice [of hospital within the United Liverpool Training School group] I was just allocated. I went to Sefton to train, I went to Alder Hey as a student and I did psychiatry. There were about 28 in my PTS group at Sefton, mostly women, five boys, only one older student, she was about 28 and we were all eighteen, there was one chap from Ghana, about half were from Liverpool the remainder came from all over the country, two Irish nurses from the south, two from the Isle of Man – which was an extension of Liverpool! Drop outs? Well two had babies and had to leave and one discontinued through lack of progress.*
>
> *I lived in at Sefton General for the first 12 weeks, then you could move home. Ward allocations were about eight weeks. My first ward was a medical ward, I did quite a lot of nights on that ward which was pretty scary for an 18 year old. There were no trained nurses on the wards at night just two students and a nursing assistant, pretty scary stuff. But night sisters were fantastic and we learned very quickly, when to call them when we needed to have a trained nurse immediately. They were very good and came round very regularly. Now when I look back it terrifies me but at the time you just knew, there was a list and they said "Do this, and ring these people", and it worked and you learned very quickly. By the end of my first year I could make decisions that were very valid, and correct, very easily.*
>
> *The uniforms were fantastic – they made you feel and look like a nurse. There was a cap that was folded in three parts which was very difficult to*

manage – mine looked like a cake – with a frill at the back. It did catch on curtains and things but you looked smart. The green dress was a denim-type material, lined inside. It was issued for you – the sewing room made sure they were the right length, and they did measure them, so many inches above the ground... also of course a white starched apron, and collars that detached so you had a clean collar every day. There is no doubt about it, you looked as if you belonged to a profession and patients loved it.

Nurses were expected to look immaculate at all times: aprons were to be changed if they became soiled while on duty. The uniform of the student nurses changed according to which year of training they were in. At the United Liverpool Hospitals, first year students had just the apron; 2nd years who had passed the Intermediate Examination had the belt and 3rd years had the belt and stripes on their epaulettes. Staff nurses were in different coloured dresses and sisters were in their traditional royal blue dresses with long sleeves which could be rolled up when working with patients. Both staff and patients knew at what stage the student nurses were in their training. This was very different to the national uniform introduced in the 1970s: the polyester cotton, throw-in-the-washing-machine dresses. For Spyropolous, this was an emotive issue:

Uniforms, I may sound like an old fuddy-duddy but... uniforms do give you that sense of security. We could not go out of the hospital in our uniforms... The only people who could wear uniforms outside of the hospital were District nurses and midwives. When I worked as a student midwife you had a gabardine mac that covered your clothing and it was very specific. Even then your uniform was washed in the hospital. You had an allocation of seven and you used a laundry pack.

Until the early 1970s general, or adult, nurse training was solely based on the apprenticeship system, with learning taking place predominantly on the wards with regular one- or two-week 'blocks' of training school-based lectures and practical instruction. Since 1924 the General Nursing Council, which later became the United Kingdom Central Council and, most recently, the Nurses and Midwives Councils' English National Board, set the State Final examinations for nurses in English hospitals. Teaching hospitals also set their own 'hospital' examinations and awarded much-coveted hospital badges which were worn with pride by their recipients. Students and pupils (those training as State Enrolled Nurses) were issued with booklets, inside which were listed the nursing tasks they were expected to become proficient in during their training. As each task was accomplished and witnessed in practice, trained staff on the wards signed them off. They also detailed the practical assessments that each student and pupil had to take on the ward at different stages of their training, observed by a nurse tutor. These were an integral part of training and had to be passed before a nurse was allowed to sit their final examination. Andrea Spyropolous remembered the process:

> *We had a little beige-coloured book which we took with us to every single placement... lists of tasks, important aspects of nursing development – taking a temperature, washing the patient, aseptic technique, doing a blood pressure... Guess you'd call that continual assessment today... a little passport. There were four areas that had to be covered: basic nursing care, performing an aseptic technique, managing a ward, and medicine administration – that was strict, every drug you gave out you had to know what it was, what was the normal dosages, how it worked, what the side-effects were, quite a lot of pharmacology but nobody ever called it that, it was called medicine administration but that's what it was in effect... really useful tools and a sense of achievement and progress... I'm a bit old fashioned, I still think that anatomy and physiology is absolutely critical to nursing. I think if you don't understand the normal you can't appreciate the abnormal. It's a fundamental, along with observation, absolutely. It was tough, it wasn't easy.*

The working lives of nurses revolve around a three-shift system – a morning start or 'early', an afternoon start or 'late' and a night shift. Start and finish times vary from hospital to hospital. There are other variants, such as long days, for example from 8am – 8pm and something called a 'split'. This starts as if on an early, then there are three or four hours off in the afternoon before returning as the day shift finishes working until the night shift starts. One thing common to all shifts is the importance of taking a 'hand-over', or ward, report from the shift going off duty. It was something that Spryopolous remembered vividly:

> *Having good ward reports was critical... when I looked back those reports covered everything – from the relatives, to the relationships, to the doctors, physio – really, really inclusive, and you had a complete picture, there wasn't anything that happened to the patient that you didn't know when you took over. It was a simple mechanism but it worked very well... We worked really, really hard but had a lot of fun. We did things you couldn't possibly do today and patients joined in the jokes. We were in Nightingale*

wards so they could see everything, they knew everything that went on. They understood the hierarchy, they knew who was important and who wasn't, so there was camaraderie with the patients as junior nurses… sending a colleague for the traditional 'long stand' outside of theatre, making diseases up so we were all scrambling trying to find out what it was. There was no internet in those days, so you couldn't check it instantly. We might spend a couple of days trying to find something that didn't exist, but there was a lot of fun… People say it must have been awful when the doctors were all in control. The truth is they were never in control, you just collaborated with them. The sisters ruled the roost on any ward, they set the scene, the tone, the climate and the culture, and if it was good it was because they were good.

Spyropoulos also recalled the powerful and lasting lessons she learned from working in Liverpool hospitals, and argues that simple tasks such as washing patients could often be as valuable to the nurse as they were to the patient:

I had some of the best moments when I was washing them because it was very intimate and they talk to you as they're going through. I learned so much about people, elderly patients, I suddenly discovered that they'd had this life that was so different to the way they presented. They were old to me, 70 was old then… and you'd have a man in his 70s and he'd share with you some of the things he'd done. Some of the stories were amazing, their memories about shipping and the docks, the children. They had lived life and they really did live life… an elderly woman, who looked like your grandmother, who suddenly told you about the things that they did when they were young. I remember one woman who had been in ENSA entertaining the troops and she was remarkable. And of course once we took an interest in her she got photographs brought in and it became part of her recovery, talking about where she'd been and maybe it gave her that inspiration to go on. … I think that [nurses today] have a lot more pressure than I had. I always felt that I was looked after and there was always somebody wiser when I was a student and I could go to them, even though they were battleaxe ward sisters they still looked after you.

During the 1970s the NHS was in chronic financial crisis. This had an immediate and very detrimental effect on the lives of many student nurses. Students who had completed their three year training, many of whom were the brightest academically – consistently at the top of their group in written assessments and predicted to pass with flying colours –

inexplicably failed their State Final examinations. Rose Mawby did her SRN training between 1972–75 at the David Lewis Northern Hospital and the Liverpool Royal but qualified as an SEN. She and her friend Ruth Oscroft both took their finals in September 1975. According to Mawby a very high proportion of her set who sat State Finals in 1975 failed. (At the same time, student nurses at Manchester Royal Infirmary who had commenced SRN training in September 1972 also suffered the shock of mass failures). The belief at the time was that it was due to the critical state of NHS funding in 1975, opportunities for employing newly-qualified SRN nurses were few and far between. Put simply, there were no jobs for trained staff on the wards of hospitals across the country. There were rumours in the student nursing community that it had been expedient (and much cheaper) for the government to continue employing third year student nurses who were waiting to re-sit their State Finals than to employ newly-qualified Staff Nurses. At best it seems with hindsight that some dubious manipulation of the pass rates went on.

Rose Mawby recalled the sense of shock she felt at the time (which was still discernible at interview nearly forty years later):

> *It was a scandal, a mass failing, I think it was a political thing because there wasn't room for everyone to be employed, no jobs. People who weren't expected to, failed, they'd been top of the group. So I took it a second time but my heart wasn't in it because I was angry. I didn't take it a third time so I automatically became a State Enrolled Nurse. I'd passed all my four practical assessments with flying colours. It was really hard for those who did pass because they were really happy but everyone else was really gutted. It was awful really, I never really came back from it to be honest.*

However, she looked back on her time at the Northern very fondly:

> *It was great… more like a family atmosphere. The Royal seemed bigger and less friendly. I lived in at the Northern. We started work at 7.30, you'd get up and walk up this long, Victorian corridor and at the end of the corridor there was a lift with metal cage doors that you pulled across, massive and spooky.*
>
> *My first ward was a surgical ward… and I was just told to go and wash an old lady… she turned the bedclothes down and she had a colostomy. I hadn't even heard of a colostomy and so I had to improvise again, it was all a bit scary… and you just learned on your feet really and you worked very, very hard… we would wash our hands all the time, and there weren't the*

germs there are now, and we were trained very well how to do everything, eventually.

On nights we got the patients up at a ridiculous hour... giving them cornflakes at 6 o'clock... because there were so many of them and so few of us, you had to start early... on days everybody who needed to, had a proper bed bath and had clean sheets. And we also did oral care in those days... in my experience patients these days don't always seem to get that care, say if you've had an operation and your mouth is dry, we used to clean people's mouths regularly, put glycerine on their lips, which they don't seem to do now. We had a lot of attention to detail on that sort of thing but we weren't very good at chatting to the patients. We weren't allowed to, you know if we had finished everything we had to do we had to go and clean a cupboard.

In 1974 when I was a 2nd year student at the Liverpool Royal Infirmary, I worked on a ward called Tropics. I nursed men who had been prisoners of war in the Far East. Some of them had leg ulcers that had never healed, others had infections and some had amoebic dysentery. I was a 20 year old and felt sad and puzzled that they were still suffering so many years after the war was over. I don't think many people were aware of their suffering.

When asked about where she and other nurses had socialised in Liverpool during their student days, Mawby vividly recalled one particular haunt, the Cabin Club, on Wood Street:

There was a black tatty door and you had to knock on the door and somebody would open it... you had to go down some very dark stairs into a very dark, tiny room and there were half beer barrels, you know great big casks that the beer was in, cut in half, seats hanging from the ceiling. And there was a tiny little restaurant with a Chinese man in and he used to deal out the plates like playing cards, throwing them on to the table in front of you and you'd get a Chinese meal. And we used to do the 'stomp', a mad dance... and we used to just have a wild time. And I think it was because we worked so hard and it was all so intense and we were young and we used to go and let off steam and have a great time.

Ruth Oscroft, another of the September 1972 intake, also recalled early memories, especially

being terrified of the ward sister, having to take off your apron when going for a break. I was unfortunate to contract impetigo on my first week on the wards. I remember stamping my feet when visiting the basement blood store at the Northern at night to frighten away the cockroaches. When the first girl from our group got married we formed an arch with polished metal bedpans for the bride and groom to walk under... Innocently, I had assumed that I would pass my finals and had my wedding organised for January 1976 and hoped to start midwifery in Chesterfield, which is where we would start our married life. I was devastated when I failed! It really came out of the blue. I left Liverpool anyway as planned and then had to arrange to re-sit my finals in Chesterfield as an external candidate, which I did and was successful.

Lesley Elliott started SRN training on 1 January 1973:

I applied to... the United Liverpool Hospitals. Then went into PTS in the Hospital College in the new Royal, for eight weeks but I was allocated to the David Lewis Northern Hospital. We actually stayed, ate and slept, at Woolton Manor but went to college daily. I started on a medical ward and the patients were very heavy and dependent – very, very seriously ill. There were armies of us, loads of staff under the direction of the trained staff and the ward sisters. We got a report first thing from night staff and sister allocated jobs to be done. So many bed-baths, washes, assisting patients, sitting them in a chair or putting them back to bed. Very repetitious and heavy work. We started about 7.20 then you had three quarters of hour for lunch, finished at 5pm that was a day shift. If you were on a split you started at the same time, finished at 12.45, and came back on again at 4:45 till 8. We did a lot of splits... I lived-in at the David Lewis Northern. That was horrendous – heavy lorries screeching to a stop outside, the whole building used to shake, so on nights you never got a full sleep.

Elliott recalled working on the round wards at the Royal.

They used to make me feel like I was on a treadmill, but what was great was from the door you could see every patient so you knew exactly if somebody needed you, or if you were required anywhere. Whereas with the long Nightingale wards I mean it was hard, especially if the curtains were pulled a bit, to see everybody to make sure everybody was okay.

These were the same round wards that Florence Nightingale had objected to when the hospital was being designed in the 1880s, as she believed they did not allow as much air circulation as the pavilion-style ward.

Maggie Hammond, who undertook her SRN training at Broadgreen between 1971 and 1974, remembers especially,

> *casualty nights... intensive care... huge responsibility as a 2nd year student... being reprimanded by Matron for having the pillow cases the wrong way round... serving dinners in the ward... watching a patient take off his oxygen and light a cigarette... first operation in the orthopaedic theatre (carpal tunnel syndrome)... having Guinness vomited all over me... gooseberries and custard, apple crumble... all the time I was training I looked forward to the day when I could wear the beautiful lilac staff nurses' uniform with the stiff cuffs and the frilly bits you put over your sleeves when you rolled them up, and the belt... our uniforms were washed and ironed for us and we changed at work; it seems wrong to me that nurses now wear their work clothes outside the hospital. I was so proud of my uniform and felt wonderfully professional when wearing it.*

District nursing

District nursing remained true to the vision of its founders, William Rathbone VI and Florence Nightingale. When the NHS was created in 1948 it was decided that the service would be managed by Local Authorities, who also provided public health services such as vaccinations and health visiting, and personal social services. This was hugely significant for the Queen's Nurses who were trained by, or under the auspices of, the Queen's Institute of District Nursing (QIDN). From 1959 the length of the district nurse training course provided by the QIDN was reduced from six to four months, with employing authorities requiring 18 months post-certificate service. The reduced period of training disadvantaged district nurses for a considerable time during a time of changing health needs and care provision. In 1968 the Panel of Assessors for the Education and Training of District Nurses (established in 1959), made up of senior district nurses and nurse tutors, took over district nurse training from the QIDN.

To those district nurses working in the new NHS, the most important thing was that they no longer had to worry about whether people could pay for nursing services as they were now free to all. Florence Nightingale fervently believed that the district nurses should not become 'alms givers': she wanted to separate the skilled women who were trained as nurses from the kind ladies who visited the homes of the poor doling out money to people in need. This central concern remained pivotal to the development of district nursing. District nurse training also reflected the critical role of public health: learning about clean water, clean air, avoiding infections, teaching people about diet and nutrition and how to look after themselves.

The 1974 reorganisation of the NHS moved the location of district nursing services from Local Authorities into the Family Practitioner branch of the NHS, where they remained until the Thatcher restructuring of the 1980s. This coincided with the creation of the Specialist Practitioner qualification which replaced the traditional district nursing training course. From the early 1990s there was another period of great change and by 2012 the district nursing qualification was no longer a prerequisite for all 'community' nursing posts. Indeed, in some parts of Britain the training of district nurses ceased altogether.

A recent campaign run by the Queens Nursing Institute, (QNI – the QIDN changed its name again in 1973) called *Right Nurse, Right Skills* focused on the skills and qualifications that are essential to good practice for those working in the community as a district nurse. Rosemary Cook, Director of the QNI, explained the confusion that has arisen:

> *Exactly what qualifications those people called 'district nurse' actually have varies enormously these days. There are nurses with no community experience who move into a community post and become a district nurse because they work on the district, but they may have no specific training for working outside hospitals... They may of course have done a variety of individual courses – there's much more commissioning of ad hoc modules and courses at university. So they'll do their prescribing training for example, and they might do something on assessment and advanced assessment and they may do something on wound care, or whatever... picking elements of the job to skill people up in. But what they're missing is that overarching understanding of [caring for] people at home.*

The profession lost over a third of trained district nurses in the decade to 2007 but the number of Health Care Assistants (HCAs) working in the community more than doubled during that period. They are not nurses, although they may have had training in various procedures and are qualified to carry out some quite technical tasks for patients. But nevertheless the anxiety is that an HCA may go in to a home and do a very good job of dressing a leg ulcer because they've been trained how to do dressings on leg ulcers, but they might not pick up and act upon other information about the health needs of that patient as a trained and experienced district nurse would do, such as an unusual smell, the ambient temperature, or relationships within the family. GPs have also increasingly employed HCAs to work in their surgeries, again to do routine tasks.

A series of reports, including specifically the *Value for Money* report published in 1992 by the NHS Executive, effectively reduced district nursing to a set of tasks such as giving injections, dressing leg ulcers, nutrition and diet. It overlooked the fundamental essence of the role, as Nightingale and Rathbone had seen it very clearly, which was that the district nursing service was a holistic approach to caring for the individual in the context of their family, home and environment; care in its broadest sense, not simply carrying out of a series of tasks. The 1999 Audit Commission report into district and community nursing was also charged with looking at the tasks district nurses were doing and ask whether the service was good value for money. Rosemary Cook described the mood within the district nursing profession in 2012:

> *The end result for district nurses has been a sense of not being valued, not being understood in the complexity of what they do, which I think is quite true – low morale and high pressure – and it has absolutely spiraled downwards. So, district nursing now is very, very diverse across the country. There are places where they're really investing in it and they really do value the title and they have people who are qualified. But there are other places where they have removed the title of district nurse from all of their community nurses, they don't want to use it. They think it's an old-fashioned title. They've got case managers, complex case managers, community staff nurses, all sorts of titles…*

The huge changes in health care from the 1970s have increased the demand for skilled health care in the home. Earlier discharge from hospital after both major and day case surgery, advances in medication and treatment regimes for housebound chronic sick patients and the inexorable rise in the elderly population, with many living to well over a hundred, have placed new burdens on district nursing. People are now much more likely to have several long-term and often complex conditions that require care. Although there are more qualified nurses working in the community than there were ten years ago, there are far more inexperienced nurses, non community-qualified nurses and even newly-qualified nurses, who go directly into community care and inevitably the skill mix is weaker. This will change further as more and more traditionally-qualified district nurses retire in the 2010s.

However, as the NHS faces its greatest change since its inception, district and community nursing may find itself in the forefront of developments, with the creation Clinical Commissioning Groups led by GPs, who often have a much better understanding of the capacity of district nursing than the former Primary Care Trusts. Rosemary Cook therefore sees this as

> *the cusp of a really exciting time for community nursing. There is potential, both with the new commissioners, who really rate the value of having this sort of service… and the opportunity to work much more closely with the patients going in and coming out [of hospital]. It could be a really good chance to integrate services in a way that we've never managed in the last 30 years.*

District nursing in Liverpool

Angela Hogg undertook her district nurse training in Liverpool in 1967 in one of the final groups to be trained by the Queen's Institute for District Nurses. She regarded the influence of the QIDN in her training as very beneficial:

> *It was very procedure-orientated, gave one a finesse in practice. Actually, if one was to make a comparison, the QNI procedures were an equivalent to the procedures performed by Royal Infirmary or Northern nurses, there was such finesse to them. These days nurses would laugh but even to opening the Gladstone bag in a certain way, unwrapping the instruments, there was a procedure to go through even for handling the instruments in the bag, standing the instruments up in the bag.*

These procedures were part of the routine that district nurses were trained in. They were used to create an air of competence and confidence from the moment that the nurse entered a patient's home. No matter what they had to do, or what they were there to confront, they at all times appeared unflappable, in charge, creating by every move and gesture a capability that in their care the patient was completely safe. Angela believes that the uniform was critical to their success:

> *We were going into homes in highly recognisable nurses uniform, not the sort of Tesco's till outfits they wear today. One would even fold the apron in a certain way to prevent contamination of the inside of the coat. The apron with bib and belt stayed on from the beginning of the day. But before you put the coat on you actually folded the apron… this part in, that part in…*

so, right and left sides to the centre, then the bottom taken up and either pinned on to the belt or tucked under the belt. It was believed that in fact any contamination on the apron, because it was folded in that way, would not contaminate the lining of the coat. Midwives folded theirs the opposite way because they were protecting the baby and mother from contamination. We were protecting ourselves because of cross infection. When one went into a house the coat, the outside, was folded in and wrapped over and the patient provided newspaper for the nurse to put it on. Everything was governed by these procedures, the whole of practice was, but I think the patients really recognised that authority. And of course we were covered in badges as well, and hats with the QIDN badge, we had an air of authority. One of the GPs used to say to me 'Oh here comes the blessed army again!' And I think patients not only respected it which they did, but also did feel quite confident that you knew what you were doing, you could help them.

Patients had to bake the dressings and we'd boil our syringes. After CSSD [Central Sterile Supplies Department] supplies came in, then we carried disposable syringes.

Angela Hogg was one of twenty district nurses covering inner city Liverpool in the 1970s, including one male nurse, Alf Summers (with perhaps one or two more men working at the district nurses' centre at Walton). She did not live-in but travelled to work from Allerton daily, as the senior superintendent Miss Basterfield, who worked with the Medical Officer of Health, did not like district nurses to work in the area in which they lived. The two main District Nursing Centres covering the city were Walton in Church Road and the Central Home in Grove Street, which covered the southern area and which was attacked and set on fire during the 1981 riots, though thankfully it was not destroyed. There were also peripheral centres in the outer suburbs, such as Deepdale, Ashcombe Road, one out at Speke which was a purpose-built home, and Rose Lane which catered for a more affluent part of Liverpool around Childwall. These were a contrast to the deprived inner city areas of Liverpool served from the Grove Street or Walton Homes.

Hogg was attached to three GPs who were all in single-handed practices quite a distance apart. She preferred to walk the district rather than cycle, looking after their patients and doing weekly clinics at each surgery for the routine things like Cytamen injections and ear syringing. Her districts were: 'Cathedral' the area around the Anglican cathedral; 'St Paul's' which covered the Dingle and was known as the 'Holy Land' because of the names of the streets which ran between Park Road and

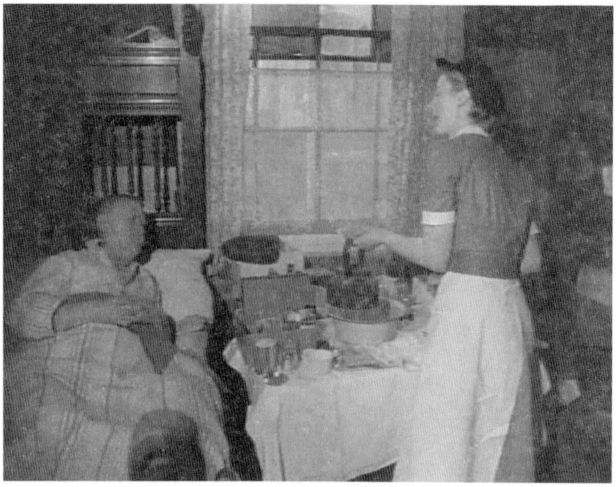

Figure 4.4 *A district nurse at work*

Mill Street; and 'Princes Park' which was the triangle of Princes Road, Upper Parliament Street and Kingsley Road. There was an awareness of the need to extend clinical nursing skills as well as looking after patients in their homes and developing skills alongside the medical practitioners. However, there was resistance to change from some GPs, who relied on district nurses to 'mop up' a wide range of issues.

Looking back on her career as a district nurse Hogg found there were one or two patients that readily came to mind:

> *The long-term patients you'd become very close to and so many were isolated. I remember one little lady, she lived in a tenement building in Liverpool 8, off Mill Street. She developed an oesophageal restriction and every morning I went in and had to boil up the oesophageal bougie in a saucepan and then once cooled I would pass this to dilate the oesophagus... she never complained. I can see her now sitting in this very poor sitting room. She had a wooden table and she sat on a dining room chair... she sat there all day. So pleasant and sweet and she just looked forward to this visit and I'd have a cup of tea with her and we'd chat about things. She lived day in, day out like that, the room was so spartan, newspaper table-cloth... she sat there with great calmness. She would absolutely depend on you and you had absolutely no facilities. Hand washing was at a cold tap.*

Even in the 1960s Liverpool still had large numbers of slum dwellings. Many of them were Victorian terraced houses that had survived the inter-war council re-housing programmes and the Blitz and there were even a few of the old court and cellar houses still inhabited. Although

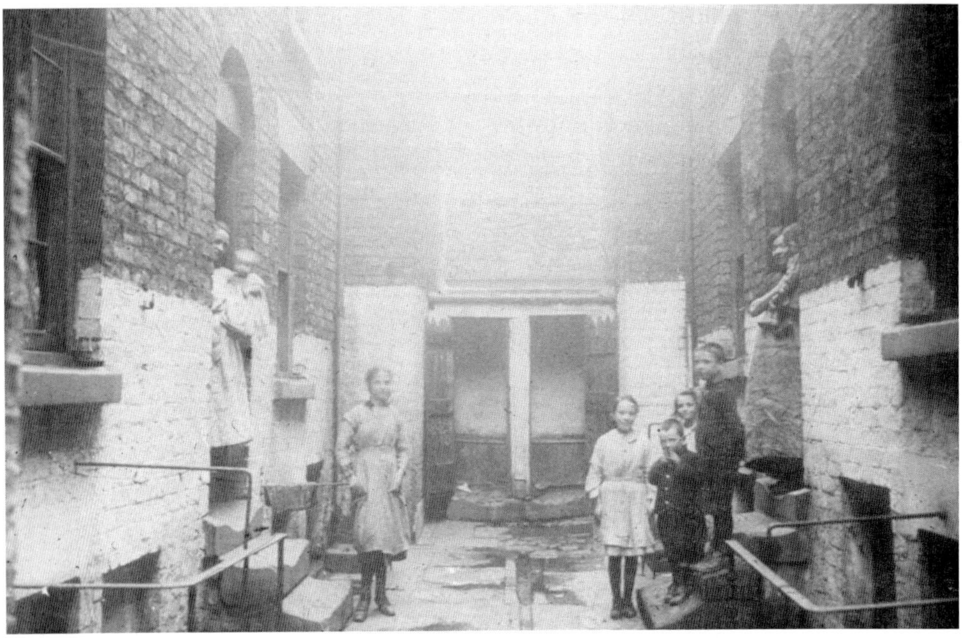

Figure 4.5 *Liverpool's court and cellar slum housing*

these housing conditions were becoming rare they stuck in the memories of many of Liverpool's district nurses. Hogg also recalled visiting a patient in the Duke Street district:

> *I went into the house [off the court] and it glowed and smelt of Mansion polish, I think it was, and there was only lino on the floor and a sideboard which had so much polish on, and it gleamed and the smell was beautiful. And a little lady sitting by the side of the coal fire and she was spotlessly clean. And I was so amazed by the difference between this external area which seemed so grubby and so awful in the sunshine and yet in this little house it was absolutely spotless.*

However, Liverpool City Council had invested heavily in the inter-war years to replace slum housing with modern homes which had amenities such as hot running water and inside WCs. Model schemes in the city centre included St Andrews Gardens and Gerard Gardens, and in the suburbs new estates were developed at Speke, Walton, Norris Green, Aintree and Kirkby. This greatly helped the work of Liverpool's district nurses. In the post-war years the city council demolished further areas of terraced housing, replacing them with less popular high-rise blocks of flats on estates such as Netherley. Although this helped to reduce overcrowding, it destroyed existing communities and created access problems, especially for the elderly and those with young children. Liverpool was again at the forefront of innovations in district nursing when it introduced a night service in 1969. Initially it was restricted to weekday nights and provided sitters and carers throughout night. Prior to this service, patients had to use the Marie Curie night service which meant paying a contribution to the charity.

After working on the district Hogg went to London to train in nurse education. She qualified as a Registered Nurse Tutor later gaining the Community Health Nurse Tutor's certificate as well, which encompassed occupational health, health visiting and district nursing. In 1972 she returned to Liverpool to work in district nurse education, becoming a Senior Nursing Officer (SNO) based at Woolton Manor's Community Health Teaching centre, before transferring with the department to the new, state-of-the-art Hospital College.

A new curriculum for district nurse education and training was implemented in 1981. It provided a six-month course followed by a three-month period of supervised practice, and was mandatory for employment as a district nurse. However, the Panel of Assessors for District Nurse Education and Training and then the new English National Board, required the transfer of the courses to Higher Education Institutions following the lead made by health visitors. Liverpool was not as progressive as some other places in making this transition partly because of organisational issues within the University of Liverpool.

It was not until 1987 that the district nurse training course was transferred from the Hospital College in the RLUH to the university's Whelan Building (the former Victorian Medical School), alongside other Professions Allied to Medicine such as physiotherapy, radiography and health visiting in the adjacent Thompson-Yates Building. This close academic environment helped to boost academic standards and foster research. Hogg recalled that,

> *it opened up a brand new world of debate and conversation that we had never had before. We were now in a position to be challenged but also to be valued for knowledge we brought… it was a great event to make that move, it was recognition.*

District nurse tutors were now also working alongside doctors in the university's Department of General Practice. Practice nursing was growing rapidly and large numbers were already employed in GPs' surgeries across the city. These were usually older married women, many of whom had been trained at the Royal who had left nursing to raise their families; now they wanted to get back into nursing but they needed jobs that would fit in with family life. Professor Ian Stanley, head of the Department of General Practice, involved district nurse tutors in developing a new curriculum and associated short training courses. Practice nurses took up the challenges of asthma care and diabetes, for which they took great deal of responsibility. GPs were enthusiastic and very supportive. They recognised that these women may have been away from nursing for some time, but that they'd been drilled so well in hospitals that they gave a tremendous range of care to patients.

Tom Donovan started his nursing in 1972 aged 18, training to be a Registered Mental Nurse (RMN) at the large psychiatric hospital at Rainhill. Once qualified he joined the United Liverpool Hospitals to do the eighteen month SRN short course and worked at Sefton General Hospital. In 1982, he started district nurse training. During his general training there had been restrictions to the patients Donovan could nurse. He was only allocated to male wards. He never worked in maternity care or child health care. However, he quickly discovered that in district nursing things varied considerably for men working in the community:

> *There were different models. In Liverpool I had a mixed case load [men, women and children] and I didn't think anything of that at all. In other towns, e.g. Wirral and Southport, there were clear gender divides, you would have a fully trained male district nurse and he'd just do catheters all day, which is just crazy. That has changed... that was a traditional model. Liverpool was far more progressive, as a male district nurse I had the same caseload as everybody else.*

Liverpool and the development of Graduate Nurse Education

While many of the older generation of trained nurses believe that their State Registered Nurse (SRN) which later changed to Registered General Nurse (RGN), or State Certified Midwife (SCM) qualifications are as good as any first degree, most knew that these qualifications had no real currency outside of nursing. Many were pleased that the academic status of nursing was subsequently raised, both in terms of the opportunities for professional development and also an acknowledgement of the knowledge that nurses acquire through the years of training and practice. Prior to the introduction of degree qualifications, in addition to SRN, RGN and SCM, state nursing qualifications included: State Enrolled Nurse (SEN) later known as Enrolled Nurse (EN), Registered Mental Nurse (RMN), Registered Sick Children's Nurse (RSCN), Registered Nurse Mental Handicap (RNMH) now known as Registered Nurse Learning Disabled (RNLD) and Registered Fever Nurse (RFN) which was discontinued in the 1960s.

The next two decades saw major changes to nurse training and education in England. The 1979 Nurses, Midwives and Health Visitors' Act recommended the move away from the apprenticeship model. The United Kingdom Central Council for Nursing, Midwifery and Health Visiting (UKCC), comprising four national boards (the English board being known as the ENB), was created to supervise nurse education and training. The move into Higher Education came as a result of the findings of the RCN's Judge Report in 1985. Nursing was now seen as highly technical and specialised and caring for the sick a marginal activity which could be carried out by HCAs largely.

Liverpool was one of the first places in Britain in which training moved from hospital-based schools of nursing into higher education institutions. In 1969 discussion began between Liverpool hospitals and the University of Liverpool's Faculty of Medicine with a view to establishing an academic Department of Nursing, headed by Liverpool-trained nurse tutor Kate Morle. The first degree course started in 1971 and it combined a Bachelor of Science degree in Life Sciences with the SRN qualification. The course ran until the late 1980s.

From as early as 1934 discussions had taken place about replacing the existing Royal Infirmary with a much larger hospital. It was to take forty years before this became a reality. While the fourth Royal was in the final planning stages, the NHS underwent its first comprehensive reorganisation, which took effect in 1 April 1974. The efficiency emphasis behind the changes mirrored the economic concerns of the period (the OPEC oil crisis and worldwide recession of the 1970s). The NHS reorganisation further intensified the trend towards managerialism. Nursing was not immune, and there were some benefits, which saw nurses given equal status alongside doctors and hospital managers in planning services. However, nursing manager roles were usually filled by male nurses, wildly out of proportion to their representation in the nursing body. The 1979 Nurses, Midwives and Health Visitors Act consolidated these changes, and brought together all aspects of nursing and health visiting to form a strong professional lobby and control over entry standards through the independent UKCC.

Another innovation in nursing practice was the role of the nurse practitioner which was developed in North America from the early 1970s, initially in response to a shortage of doctors in the USA. Nurses worked closely with the medical team, learning how to take histories and doing much of the routine pre- and post-operative patient care especially in response to the rise in day case work. In the early 1980s the first nurse practitioners in the UK worked in GP surgeries, closely supported by the doctors and taking on such work as diagnosis, treatment and referral to consultants. Many former 'treatment room' nurses trained as nurse practitioners often becoming the first point of contact for patients. Out of this grew the role of the specialist nurses who developed expertise in a particular field, for example diabetes or community nursing.

The UKCC published Project 2000 in 1986. This tried to end the reliance of hospitals on the labour of student nurses, and to shift nursing education away from wards and into colleges. Project 2000 had replaced the old apprenticeship State Registration training and created the new Registered General Nurse (RGN). For the first time student nurses were not to be part of the ward staff – they were now supernumerary. It also saw the end of SEN training which put a much greater reliance on largely untrained nursing auxiliaries to do the basic nursing care. However, while the new RGNs were awarded a diploma in higher education and a professional nursing qualification, the emphasis on the theoretical aspects of nursing were to have a detrimental effect on the acquisition of practical skills and training.

In 1992 the new Liverpool John Moores University (or LJMU, formerly Liverpool Polytechnic) started the first diploma-level course. The Liverpool School of Nursing and Midwifery had moved the nurse training schools formerly based at Broadgreen General Hospital, the Royal Liverpool Hospital, Alder Hey Children's Hospital and Liverpool Maternity Hospital, to LJMU. Its Department of Nursing also combined with Central Mersey College, bringing together Whiston Hospital, St Helen's Hospital, Warrington General, Winwick and Rainhill Hospitals' nursing and midwifery training schools. Liverpool John Moores University Faculty of Health's Nursing Department has become the major provider of midwifery, adult, child and mental health nurse education in Merseyside with over 900 pre-registration nursing students undertaking professional programmes at LJMU at any one time.

Tom Donovan joined the University of Liverpool's Department of

Nursing in 1998 to deliver the oncology option of the Bachelor of Nursing with Honours (BN Hons) programme:

> *We were part of the 1971 off-shoot, the experimental group, which started small, we only recruited about ten nurses a year... the entry criteria were much higher and there were fewer candidates with those qualifications. A lot of people couldn't see a need for the degree and they didn't make the connection, because nursing was based on a traditional model of apprenticeship, nursing knowledge was gained through experience rather than research. People couldn't see the reason for an academic approach to nursing, couldn't see a need for nursing research. That came much, much later on.*

The University of Liverpool's Department of Nursing was founded on the idea of developing nursing knowledge through research. Initially the degree lasted four years: nurses would qualify in Year 3 as a Registered Nurse and then go immediately into an area of specialist practice, either district nursing or health visiting. Changes to nursing regulations in 2000 altered it to a three-year degree but it retained the title of Bachelor of Nursing because it was important that it had distinct identity as a nursing degree.

By 2012 the University of Liverpool enrolled around 40 students a year, up to a maximum of 44, a relatively small number compared to other local universities such as Liverpool John Moores, Edge Hill and Chester who have recruited two to three hundred at a time, sometimes twice a year. Although the student numbers on the University of Liverpool degree course has remained around 40, the numbers of applicants has exceeded 1,000. Concerns that degree-qualified nurses would wish to move away from clinical practice and into research have proved unfounded. The University of Liverpool course has attracted the majority of its students from outside Liverpool, but they usually stay to work in the city after qualifying.

The Fourth Liverpool Royal Infirmary

The first part of the new Royal to open had been the Hospital College in 1968. It took much longer for the wards to transfer into the new building, bringing together staff from the Royal, the David Lewis Northern, the Royal Southern as well as many other smaller hospitals such as St Paul's Eye Hospital in Old Hall Street. Gradually these hospitals closed – the David Lewis Northern in 1978, the Royal Southern in 1979, St Paul's Eye Hospital in 1992 and Mill Road in 1993 – and the buildings were eventually demolished. These institutions were sadly missed by many of those who had worked in them. The wards in the new hospital eventually began receiving patients in 1978. Many nurses recalled the process of transferring across the road from the old Royal to the new. It took time for staff to get used to the new layout of the wards which were separated into four and six-bedded bays. Andrea Spyropoulos:

> *It seemed fantastic... the rooms looked very spacious, we had more than one bath, that was luxury, and we had shower rooms. But... we realised very quickly the design (from the 60s), the concept, was out of date with modern nursing. The biggest issue was the staffing. I couldn't quite work out why I needed more staff when I had fewer patients, because the ward was smaller. And it was just because the patients couldn't see you... they could be bleeding to death or they might want a newspaper... so we were constantly doing more leg work and staffing levels had to increase... But it was exciting, it looked fabulous, you've got to put it in the context then... it was brand new, everything worked and it was big, it was pretty fab...*

Palliative Care and the Liverpool Care Pathway

The hospice movement and the specialty of palliative care were founded by Cicely Saunders. The first British hospice for the care of the dying, St Christopher's, was opened in Sydenham, south west London in 1967. Having first trained as a nurse during the war years, then a social worker and finally as a doctor, Saunders gave her working life to alleviating suffering and indignity at the end of life. She spearheaded the movement towards managing terminal pain so that patients could find peace in the final stage of their lives. Saunders believed that every person is an individual to the end of life. She revolutionised the way society views the process of dying by bringing dignity, respect and humanity to the care of not only the dying but also their relatives.

In 1911 Douglas Macmillan, having witnessed his father's distressing death from cancer, founded the Society for the Prevention and Relief of Cancer. His aim was to help others in a similar situation by supplying information and encouraging education about the disease to help patients and their relatives, doctors and the public. In the hundred years since it was founded his charity, now known as Macmillan Cancer Support, has grown into one of the most prominent cancer charities in the country. Fundraising supports the training of specialist Macmillan nurses who work in hospitals and the community.

Anita Roberts started her training in September 1976 doing the combined Registered Sick Children's Nurse and State Registered Nurse course qualifying in 1980. She stayed in adult nursing as a staff nurse on a gynaecology ward at the new Royal, where she first confronted the difficulties of managing the nursing needs of often young, terminally-ill women on a busy acute ward:

> *I found it very hard, we were similar in age, I didn't know what to say... there was no palliative care at the Royal at that time... nothing had prepared me for this, no help, no support for the patient.*

In 1985, after five years' post-registration work in gynae, Roberts took a job at Sunnybank, the Marie Curie Home for the terminally ill in Woolton, to develop her skills in the care of the dying. Initially she found the change of environment coming from the new, state-of-the-art Liverpool Royal to what had formerly been a residential house then a Police orphanage, very difficult:

> *It was like stepping back into Victorian times. The staff were mainly care assistants with a few enrolled nurses and RGNs. There were no basins in bedrooms so you had to go down the corridor to wash your hands, equipment was old fashioned, nothing up-to-date. I got used to it and new ways of working and started to see things differently. Matron was very progressive with lots of ideas, the management team were sent on courses, she was keen to update the organisation... there was a 'Dunkirk' spirit, battling to modernise.*
>
> *I remember the first syringe driver, we used it on a lady who was very ill. It was a wind-up syringe driver with a big brass key; a 50ml syringe was put into the wooden casing and it ran for 12 hours... ticking like a clock it delivered the dose continually. Compared to now it was very unsophisticated, very basic, but it did the job. By degrees we learned, we improved; as palliative care has developed so has our ability to keep people comfortable and symptom-controlled.*

A massive fund-raising scheme enabled Sunnybank to be re-built as a state-of-the-art hospice – the Liverpool Marie Curie Cancer Care Centre – in 1993. Among the many innovations in the new centre there was Day Care (started while at the old Home) as well as a new philosophy of discharging patients, which previously had seemed impossible for the terminally ill. But once treatment and particularly pain relief were under control patients could manage at home for increasing periods of time. This was also driven by the fact that the Centre was often full and lacked the space for new admissions. It also facilitated the creation of an outpatients' clinic to monitor progress of patients while in the community. Other innovations in the palliative care service, as it was increasingly known, included a Community Liaison Service, with two nurses who visited people at home to assess pre-admission. The charity also developed a bank of nurses providing a sitting service with patients in their own homes overnight. Roberts remembers it as,

> *a period of camaraderie, all pulling together, a new era with a new building. We started to employ doctors, Dr (later Professor) John Ellershaw was appointed as a consultant, the first consultant role. We had already developed links with the Pain Relief Foundation at Walton before we moved into new building; Dr Chris Wells used to come over and see patients with uncontrolled pain problems. We got involved in research and employed a research nurse and developed an education service, we had a tutor.*

These developments were followed by education links, as student and qualified nurses, medical students and doctors all wanted to learn about palliative care. Roberts moved into education working with Susie Wilkinson (who ran oncology courses at Manchester's Christie Hospital) to devise and run courses for several years. It was a period of rapid change and development:

> *There were no clinical nurse specialists when I had worked at the Royal. Macmillan Nursing were very active in establishing these roles, pump-priming staff posts for the first three years of service on the proviso that the Trust would fund them thereafter. Deborah Murphy eventually became the Clinical Nurse Specialist in palliative care. When Dr Ellershaw was appointed his contract gave him sessions at the Royal. Now that team has grown with Deborah and Professor Ellershaw managing the Directorate of Palliative care. Professor Ellershaw has also become Assistant Director of the End of Life Care programme, working with Mike Richards at national level and linked to the Liverpool Care Pathway.*

In the early 1990s at the Royal 'pathways' were devised for various medical conditions, including stroke and hip fractures, co-ordinated by Sue Overill. Despite initial reservations, the palliative care team soon realised there would be many benefits to training ward staff to effectively manage uncomplicated, expected deaths, using the 'pathway' philosophy. This became known as the Liverpool Care Pathway for the Dying Patient (LCP). As word got out that the LCP was a really helpful process, the team was awarded Beacon status by the NHS which provided funding to disseminate it through study days, attended by clinical staff from across Britain. However, the team was very aware that great care had to be taken in implementing the LCP. It was not just a document that was sent out to wards, but a whole way of thinking that required preparing the environment before implementation. The Liverpool staff soon recognised its potential as part of a continuous quality improvement programme.

In 2004 the National End of Life Care programme was established. The Liverpool Care Pathway for the Dying Patient was recognised in NICE (National Institute for Clinical Excellence) guidance and also in documents from the Department of Health, as a key end of life care tool. There was greater demand for study days to introduce it and the team went all over the country at the request of health authorities. As it was increasingly used there was an awareness of the need for organisations to prepare the ground, putting the policies and resources in place, but also there had to be monitoring. It took on average a minimum of six months for organisations to prepare the environment. By 2012 version twelve of the LCP was being implemented after an extensive two year consultation and feedback from patients' groups, clinicians and voluntary organisations, such as churches, with an interest in the care of the dying.

Developing effective communication skills training is a fundamental part of these developments and Roberts and others have been instrumental in devising specific courses for senior nursing staff. Nurses have always been taught how to listen to patients but it is only since the 1970s that they have been taught how to 'talk' to them.

After six years working as a district nurse Tom Donovan began training as a Macmillan Nurse in Southport. He recalled how he had first learned of this new specialist field of nursing:

> *The first inkling I had of palliative care I was working on a surgical ward and talking to one of the then clinical teachers. She was a nun, and she gave me a little leaflet about St Christopher's Hospice and said this is what they're doing here. And it really made me think about the dying patient as part of a group of people needing very, very special care. And that really sparked my interest so when I got the chance to work in palliative care I*

jumped at it. I did that for ten years. There was very little training for this new specialism, nobody knew what was needed. The only recognised training were two ENB courses, 931 and 285 concerned with Care of Dying Patient.

In palliative care, interestingly, Southport [at first] was more ahead of the game than Liverpool, Liverpool's palliative care was very, very limited. We didn't know how to manage pain. Liverpool led the way appointing the first hospital-based Macmillan Nurse at the Royal.

Cardiology and intensive care nursing

Another area where there was pioneering work going on was in Cardiology at Sefton General, which in the 1960s and 1970s was the Regional Cardiology Centre. Margaret Bodha had trained at Sefton from 1960 to 1964. While awaiting her State final results in late 1964 she was working on the cardiology ward when she was invited to join a new, experimental team on the ward. The Centre had joined forces with the Hammersmith Hospital in London to pilot the first Coronary Care Unit in the country. Sister Alice Thomas was recruited from Mossley Hill Hospital to run the unit and Bodha was invited to join her, along with an SEN and a few part-time staff nurses. Initially they had two adjacent side rooms on the corridor leading to the ward, which had been set aside for the purpose. Patients were admitted according to strict criteria, for example, it had to be their first heart attack. Bodha clearly remembered those early days:

It was very rudimentary, I had no specific training and learned on the job. There was a connecting door between the two rooms and our desk was positioned near the doorway so we had sight of both patients. It was almost 1:1 nursing. We explained in detail everything we were doing which was a new approach. The ECG machines were on the bedside lockers, an oxygen cylinder stood beside each bed and we had a 'crash' [resuscitation] trolley close at hand. There were lots of consultants, two I can readily recall are Dr Norman Coulshed and Dr Charles McKendrick but they were all very involved in the detail and we had lots of visiting doctors in the early years.

In 1969 the unit, with Sister Joyce Fairbrother now leading the nursing team, moved into the first purpose-built six-bed Coronary Care Unit in the country. Equipment was becoming more and more sophisticated and much of it was wall-mounted at the bedside with oxygen also now

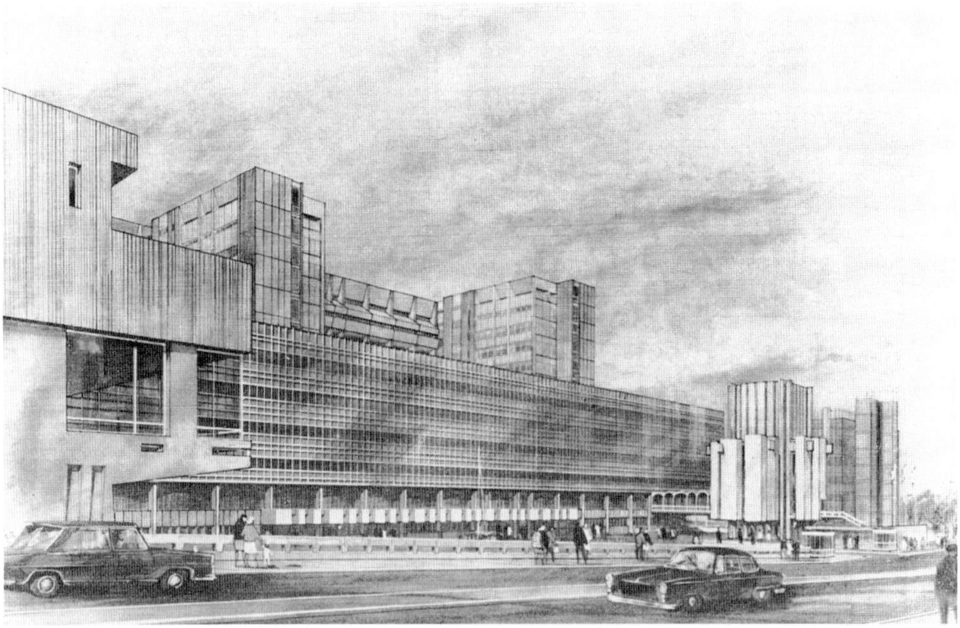

Figure 4.6 *Architect's drawing of the fourth Royal, 1967*

piped and there was a central console equipped with monitors from where staff could closely observe the condition of each patient. In 1987 the whole department moved across to the new regional cardiothoracic centre at Broadgreen Hospital.

The Nursing Process and recent experiences

Veronica Savage was 21 when she commenced her RGN training at the Royal in 1980. She had previously trained as a librarian but decided she needed to do something more fulfilling:

> *… I remember one tutor that really stands out, her name was Mrs G and I'll never forget her biology lesson as I have an image of her pretending to be the fallopian tubes and the ovaries, standing there with her arms stretched out and fingers fluttering, acting the fallopian tubes, hilarious! My first ward was an orthopaedic ward, I was working with a Chinese girl called Sue… and we had our first death in the first week. Lovely sister, authoritarian, can't recall her name… I thought I'd be frightened of death but the staff were really good nurses, taught us to be respectful, gave us the*

capability to be able to deal with anyone who had died. I learnt it on that first ward, she was an amazing trainer. Never forget the way they closed the doors on the ward, it was polite, respectful, everywhere was closed, afterwards sister took us into her office to see how we were, she was very good… She said to us that death is part of life, it's a cycle and as nurses we had a very important role… hard work orthopaedics, but enjoyable… once the patients had their fracture repaired they were healthy, I remember the camaraderie of the men, lots of laughter. The Nursing Process hadn't come in, we were given bays to look after, a 6-bed bay and a 4-bed bay… the new Royal it was all bays, you were allocated which ones to work in and you were responsible for everyone in them…

Gail Lowther started her training in March 1992 in one of the last intakes of the basic RGN training course at LJMU before the start of the Project 2000 diploma course. Qualifying in 1995 she was required to undertake a 'top-up' course to attain her diploma in line with the new qualifications. While doing this Lowther staffed on an acute orthopaedic trauma ward at the Royal for two years before moving on to the Sir Alfred Jones Memorial Hospital, a former Cottage Hospital, in Garston to work on a new intermediate care project:

The Sir Alfred Jones was lovely, a wonderful building I think it was built to serve the docks. … it served the local community and there was a minor injuries unit and GPs could admit to the unit so we didn't only take patients from the Royal. I went there in April 1997… had two-and-a-half wonderful years working in the new Intermediate Care Unit which had just been set up by Trish Bennett. It was ground-breaking at the time… designed to get people out of hospital quicker, provide a rehabilitation service closer to home that was less hospital-based and institutionalised, low-key and friendly, while being nurse-led. It was actually one of the first nurse-led units in the country, there were a couple of others that were used as the template to set it up.

Lowther was later funded to undertake the Community Specialist Practitioner degree, full time for one year, specialising in district nursing.

Paediatric nursing was another of the specialist degree courses. Kate Knight started this at Liverpool John Moores University (LJMU) in September 1998. She recalled the early days of her training:

What an exciting time. We were one of the earlier cohorts of degree students with only ten in the group… What a fantastic place to train and to be

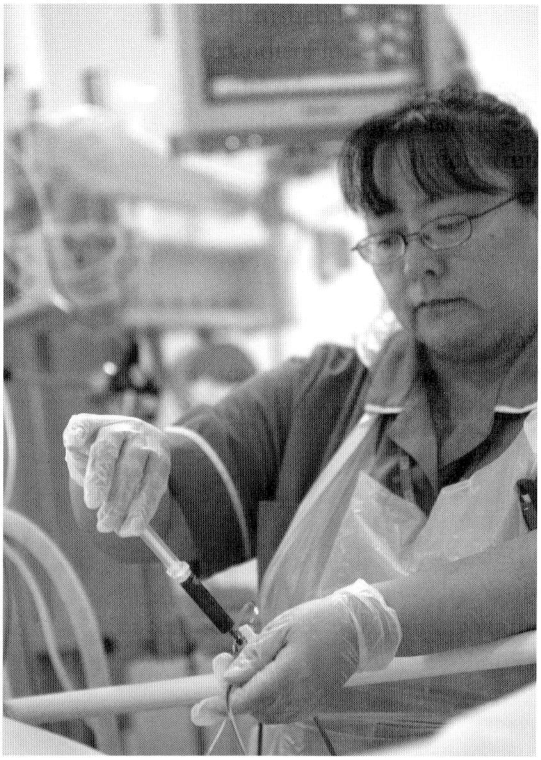

Figure 4.7 *Nurse working at the Royal Liverpool Hospital (courtesy of Royal Liverpool and Broadgreen University Hospital Trust archives)*

> *part of such history. Many of my family and friends reassured me that to study and live in Liverpool would be one of the best experiences of my life as the people are so welcoming and friendly. How true that was and I have never left! Throughout my training and career so far nursing has allowed me to meet many children, young people and families who I have been privileged to care for.*

Craig Simon graduated from the University of Liverpool in 2006 with BN Hons. He was awarded the Mary Jones and the Rebecca Haynes Awards for his achievements in training. He went on to become Charge Nurse on the Immunology Day Care Ward at the Royal. His recommendation to new trainees, based on his experience, was to befriend the Health Care Assistants (HCAs):

> *They are key to telling you how the ward is run, the routine; the HCA you turn to for the basics like bed-bathing the patient. In my first year really the key was to talk to the patients, being supernumerary, using that time to talk, finding out their stories, really important I think... it's just*

about making the most of those years training because when you qualify as a nurse, with the pressures of the current healthcare system and the way that nursing is now, you just don't get that time.

I certainly think there is such a thing as a 'Scouse' patient… doing the training through the University of Liverpool you get to experience all the different hospitals in the region. So you see the Wirral hospitals and Wirral patients, you see the St Helens and the Whiston patients, and then you've got the Royal and the Liverpool patients… if I was to sum up what a Liverpool patient was, it would be someone who was able to get across their personality.

There is definitely a strong community spirit. And you get certain areas and patients who have lived in the same street for 50 or 60 years, they've seen so much… despite whatever they're going through, despite how ill they may be, they'll still have funny tales to tell, or they'll still manage to crack a joke. I think the sense of humour of Scouse patients is second to none really. And that was the attraction of wanting to work in the Royal.

And finally mature student, Kelly Chantrill, who hopes to graduate later this year. She started the Bachelor of Nursing course at the University of Liverpool in 2009 and had this to say about studying and working in Liverpool:

I've worked at Arrowe Park, Royal Liverpool and Whiston and have enjoyed all aspects of my training. I don't want to leave! I feel nursing is seen as a valuable vocation but it is understaffed, overworked and underappreciated, but that it is generally accepted that this is the case most of the time… [Most patients are] extremely grateful and are respectful towards nurses and happy to have students learn. Nursing is a valuable vocation and I can't wait to begin my own career. The University of Liverpool has offered me a fabulous experience in a lively and reputable university. The nursing staff are so approachable and no issue is too small to ask them about. They offer support and friendship and are an asset to the university.

Conclusion

FOR NEARLY three hundred years Liverpool has been a pioneering force in healthcare. From the first voluntary hospital in the city, the Liverpool Infirmary, on Shaw's Brow in 1745, to finalising plans for the fifth Royal Infirmary adjacent to the existing hospital on Prescot Street, Liverpool has sought to provide the best care for its people.

Liverpudlians have taken a leading role in developing health services for the city. Individuals such as William Henry Duncan, who, in 1847, was appointed the Medical Officer of Health for Liverpool, the first such appointment in the country; and William Rathbone VI, the founder of district nursing and the first training school and home for nurses outside of London in 1859 and 1862 respectively. By the late 1850s Rathbone's desire to change and improve the quality of life for the town's sick poor led him to seek the advice and support of Florence Nightingale, then the foremost advocate of professional nursing in the country. They formed a remarkable partnership lasting until Rathbone's death in 1902, which changed nursing in Britain and around the world.

Since those early years of the founding of organised nurse training and its rapid spread from Liverpool to other provincial towns across the country in the late nineteenth century, Liverpool has led the way in the development of nurse training and excellence in practice. From the second half of the twentieth century onwards, in such diverse areas of care as midwifery and the management of pain during childbirth to the new discipline of Palliative Care and the development of the Liverpool Care Pathway for the care of the dying, Liverpool nurses have been at the forefront of new ideas and practices to alleviate suffering.

This book records the experiences and memories of some of Liverpool's nurses past and present. They have helped to bring to life both nursing in hospitals and in the community in doctors' surgeries and in people's homes across Liverpool, over the past sixty years. Former midwife, Lorna Muirhead, was one who welcomed the fact that,

> *the status [of nursing] has been raised... the apprentice model had a lot to commend it as does the academic model, nursing has changed dramatically.*

Liverpool again was one of the early pioneers in developing the degree programme of study for nursing. However, in recent times nursing nationally has come in for criticism mainly for not having enough qualified nurses working at the bedside. Andrea Spyropoulos, President of the Royal College of Nursing, has reflected on some of the reasons for this.

> *A lot of things have happened in nursing that's had an impact on public perception and there's a lot of media reporting of poor nursing practice... the backlash is that nurses are falling out of favour with the public. The majority of nurses that I see are still delivering fantastic care, are still working more hours than they're paid, are still going the extra mile.*
>
> *I think the public are different. I think they're much more vocal. We keep telling the public they've got rights [but] we don't give them any responsibilities to go with the rights. And their expectation of nurses is different to the expectation [of] the government... [it looks] at nursing being delivered by assistants. If you look at the ratios and skill mixes they've changed quite dramatically. We've now got very high levels of health care assistants and low levels of trained nurses... So I think it's tough for young nurses because it's not clear what is required of them.*

Tom Donovan, former Director of the University of Liverpool's Department of Nursing, made this observation:

> *We should be thinking more now about the patient's experience of health-care and the relationships that professionals make with patients... I think we've probably got more nurses than we've ever had... I think the pressures they're under are different, the job they have to do is different, and the amount of paperwork they have to do is different, and all that is taking them away from patients.*

Tony Bell, former chief executive of the Royal Liverpool and Broadgreen University Hospital Trust, whose idea it was to mark the 150th anniversary by commissioning this book, reflected:

> *I think what stood out to me about Liverpool [is that] we're all part of the history. We didn't just have the association with Florence Nightingale, we had William Rathbone VI. Liverpool has a lot to be proud of... particularly nursing, in the community and in the acute sector. In Liverpool I've always felt a really strong connection to my roots as a nurse, irrespective of where I trained, because of its association with these people, these pioneers in nursing.*

From the first intake of 20 nurses into the Liverpool training school in 1862 to those who have graduated this year from both the University of Liverpool's and Liverpool John Moores University's schools of nursing, many thousands of nurses have been trained in Liverpool over the past 150 years. The city continues to produce nurses committed to the highest standards of care for their patients wherever they may nurse them. Undoubtedly Liverpool is a special place and nursing in Liverpool was, and still is, a very special thing to do.

Sources and Additional Reading

A. R. Allan, *Sources for the History of Nursing in Liverpool* (University of Liverpool, Archives Unit, 1995).

B. Abel-Smith, *A history of the nursing profession* (London, Heinemann, 1960).

M. Baly, *Nursing and Social Change* (London, Heinemann, 1980).

M. Baly, *A History of the Queens Nursing Institute* (London, Croom Helm, 1987).

T. Bickerton, *A Medical History of Liverpool from the earliest days to the year 1920* (London, Murray 1936).

M. Bostridge, *Florence Nightingale* (London, Penguin, 2009).

C. Brewer, *A Brief History of the Liverpool Royal Infirmary 1887–1978* (Liverpool, Liverpool Area Health Authority, 1980).

M. Currie, *Fever Hospitals and Fever Nurses A British Social History of Fever Nursing: A National Service* (Abingdon, Routledge, 2005).

R. Dingwall, A. M. Rafferty, C. Webster, *An Introduction to the Social History of Nursing* (London, Routledge, 1988).

G. Hardy, *William Rathbone and the early history of District Nursing* (Ormskirk, Hesketh, 1980).

S. McGann, A. Crowther, R. Dougall, *A History of the RCN 1916–1990* (Manchester University Press, 2009).

F. Nightingale, *Organisation of nursing in a large town* (Liverpool and London: A. Holden and Longman, Green, Reader and Dyer, 1865).

E. F. Rathbone, *William Rathbone: a Memoir* (London, Macmillan, 1905).

G. Rivett, *From Cradle to Grave: Fifty years of the NHS* (London, Kings Fund, 1998).

M. Stacey, *The Sociology of Health and Healing* (London, Unwin Hyman, 1988).
P. Starkey, *Nursing memories: from probationers to professors* (Liverpool, National Museums and Galleries on Merseyside, 1994).
L. Twining, *Deaconesses for the Church of England: also a paper on the supervision and training of workhouse girls* (London, Bell and Daldy, 1860).
R. White, *Social Change and the Development of the Nursing Profession* (London, Kimpton, 1978).
C. Woodham Smith, *Florence Nightingale* (London, Constable, 1950).

Reports and Articles

J. Draper, R. Watson, 'Cadets and nursing students: same destination – different route', *Journal of Advanced Nursing*, 2002; 40(4): 449–456.
R. Huntsman, M. Bruin, C. Gibbon, 'A School for Nurses Founded in Liverpool in 1829', *Medical Historian, Bulletin of the Liverpool Medical History Society*, 2002–03; 14: 44–61.
C. Jones 'The Foundation of the Royal Liverpool Hospital Training School for Nurses 1862 History and Curriculum', accepted for publication in 2013 edition of *Medical Historian, Bulletin of the Liverpool Medical History Society.*
Leeds NHS Executive, 'The Nursing Skill-Mix in the District nursing Service' (1992).
Queens Nursing Institute, *Nursing People at Home* (November 2011).
S. Sheard, 'A Creature of its time: the critical history of the creation of the British NHS', *Michael Quarterly*, 2011; 8: 428–41.
J. Stewart, 'Ideology and Process in the Creation of the British National Health Service', *Journal of Policy History*, 2002; 14(2): 114–34.

Index

Note: Entries in bold refer to illustrations